SUNKISSED WELLNESS

The Natural Power of the Sun for
Mind and Body

WAYNE E. SMITH

ISBN: 978-1-965937-18-1 (Hardcover)
ISBN: 978-1-965937-17-4 (Paperback)
ISBN: 978-1-965937-19-8 (ePub)

Cover design by Eswari Kamireddy
Edited by Eswari Kamireddy
Interior design by Eswari Kamireddy

"Sunlight is the life-force of the world, feeding every leaf, flower, and spirit it touches."

— Anonymous

Contents

Preface   1

CHAPTER 1: The History of Sunlight and Human Health   3

Introduction to the Role of Sunlight in History   3

Sun Worship and Ancient Healing Practices   5

Scientific Discovery of Sunlight's
Benefits: From Heliotherapy to Modern Understanding of
Sunlight's Biological Effects   7

Conclusion: The Continuing Evolution of Sunlight Science   11

CHAPTER 2: Vitamin D – The Sunshine Vitamin   13

How Sunlight Stimulates Vitamin D
Production: The Skin's Role in Synthesizing Vitamin D   13

Benefits of Vitamin D: Bone Health, Immune System
Function, Mood Regulation   16

Conclusion: The Multifaceted Benefits of Vitamin D   18

Sunscreen Use: Balancing Protection and
Vitamin D Production   20

Conclusion: Addressing Modern Vitamin D Deficiency   23

CHAPTER 3: Sunlight and Mental Well-Being   25

The Connection Between Sunlight and Serotonin:
How Sunlight Boosts Serotonin and Affects Mood   25

Tackling Seasonal Affective Disorder (SAD):
Understanding Reduced Sunlight and the Benefits of
Light Therapy   27

The Role of Sunlight in Reducing Stress and
Anxiety: Exploring the Calming Effects
of Natural Light on Mental Health   29

CHAPTER 4: Circadian Rhythms and Sleep Regulation   **33**

How Sunlight Sets Your Internal Clock: The Relationship
Between Morning Sunlight and Circadian Rhythm   33

The Importance of Morning Exposure to
Sunlight: How Early Sunlight Improves Sleep Quality   36

Overcoming Sleep Disorders with Light Therapy:
How Light Exposure Can Combat Insomnia and
Other Sleep-Related Issues   40

CHAPTER 5: Sunlight and Skin Health   **45**

Sunlight as Therapy for Skin Conditions:
How Moderate UV Exposure Benefits
Psoriasis, Eczema, and Acne   45

Understand Phototherapy, which is the
therapeutic use of UV light in treating
various skin disorders.   49

Balancing Skin Health and Protection:
The Need for Safe Sun Exposure and
the Risks of Overexposure   50

CHAPTER 6: Boosting the Immune System with Sunlight   **55**

The Role of Sunlight in Immune Function:
How Sunlight Activates T-Cells and Strengthens
the Immune Response   55

Sunlight, Autoimmune Disorders, and Inflammation:
Exploring the Relationship Between Sunlight,
Vitamin D, and Reduced Inflammation in
Autoimmune Conditions   58

Seasonal Illnesses and Sunlight Deficiency:
Why We Tend to Get Sicker in Winter
When Sunlight Exposure is Lower   62

CHAPTER 7: Sunlight's Impact on Cardiovascular Health   **67**

Sunlight and Blood Pressure: How UV Rays
Release Nitric Oxide, Leading to Vasodilation and
Lower Blood Pressure   67

Reduced Cardiovascular Risks: Understanding
the Link Between Regular Sun Exposure and Lowered Risk of
Heart Attacks and Strokes   71

Exploring Sunlight's Role in Metabolic Health:
How Sunlight Can Reduce the Risk of
Diabetes and Metabolic Syndrome   75

**CHAPTER 8: The Importance of Sunlight for Children and
Adolescents**   **81**

Supporting Healthy Development: The Role of Sunlight in
Bone Growth, Mental Health, and Immune
Development in Children   81

Vitamin D Deficiency in Childhood:
The Rise of Rickets and Other Health Issues
Due to Lack of Sunlight   85

Encouraging Outdoor Play for Healthy Growth:
How Outdoor Activities in Natural Light
Contribute to Overall Well-Being   90

CHAPTER 9: Sunlight and Aging Gracefully   **95**

The Role of Sunlight in Healthy Aging:
How Adequate Sunlight Supports Strong Bones,
a Healthy Immune System, and Mental Sharpness   95

Preventing Osteoporosis and Cognitive Decline:
The Importance of Sunlight for Elderly Individuals   98

Moderate Sun Exposure for Longevity:
Studies Linking Regular, Moderate Sun Exposure
to Increased Lifespan and Quality of Life   101

**CHAPTER 10: Practical Ways to Safely Incorporate Sunlight
into Your Life   105**

Summary of Balance: 108

Recommended Products: 112

Conclusion: Embracing the Healing Power of Sunlight
Summary of the Benefits of Sunlight on Holistic Health   116

Practical Tips for Daily Sunlight Exposure   118

Final Thoughts on Harnessing Nature's Gift:
Recognizing Sunlight as a Natural,
Accessible Tool for Boosting Health, Energy, and Happiness   120

Afterword   123

Preface

Sunlight is a powerful force that has shaped life on Earth for millions of years. Its benefits are vast, from nourishing plants to providing warmth and light. But most fascinating is sunlight's profound impact on our physical and mental health. In a world where many of us spend most of our days indoors, understanding the delicate balance between reaping the benefits of sunlight and protecting ourselves from its potential dangers is more important than ever.

This book, *Sunkissed Wellness: The Natural PowerofThe Sun for Mind and Body,* is structured to provide a comprehensive understanding of the intricate relationship between sunlight, skin health, and well-being. It is designed for anyone seeking to understand better how to enjoy the advantages of moderate sun exposure while minimizing the risks of overexposure—such as sunburn, premature aging, and skin cancer.

We delve into the fascinating therapeutic uses of sunlight for skin conditions like psoriasis, eczema, and acne, shedding light on how moderate UV exposure can help alleviate these chronic conditions. But with every benefit comes a potential cost, and we explore in detail the strategies for protecting ourselves from the dangers of excessive UV radiation. This book not only highlights the role of phototherapy in controlled medical settings but also equips you with practical advice for maintaining a healthy balance between sunlight exposure and skin protection in everyday life, ensuring you are well-prepared to make informed decisions about sun exposure.

The goal of *Sukissed Wellness* is simple: to empower you with knowledge. Whether you enjoy spending time outdoors, manage a skin condition, or seek to improve your overall well-being, this book provides evidence-based insights into how sunlight affects your body and how you can make informed decisions about sun exposure. Remember, the key to reaping the benefits of sunlight while protecting your skin is knowledge and informed decision-making.

Let this guide be a source of clarity in understanding the power of sunlight. By respecting its strengths and recognizing its risks, we can enjoy the many benefits of the sun while safeguarding our health for years to come.

1

The History of Sunlight and Human Health

Introduction to the Role of Sunlight in History

From the dawn of civilization, humanity has recognized the sun as a powerful force that provides light and warmth and influences health and well-being. Ancient cultures revered the sun, intertwining its life-giving energy with their spiritual beliefs, health practices, and daily rituals. In societies like the Egyptians, Greeks, and Romans, sunlight was seen as a source of survival and a tool for healing and vitality.

The Egyptians and Sun Worship

The sun was central to religious beliefs and health practices in ancient Egypt. The Egyptians worshipped Ra, the sun god, who was considered the giver of life and controlled the cycle of birth, death, and rebirth. Sunlight was seen as divine energy capable of sustaining life and promoting physical and spiritual health. Temples were designed to allow the sun's rays to penetrate sacred spaces, and some healing practices involved exposing the body to the sun to harness its therapeutic properties.

The Greeks: Sun as Medicine

The Greeks also recognized the therapeutic value of sunlight. The physician Hippocrates, often called the "Father of Medicine," advocated using sunlight in healing. Greek medical practices involved "heliotherapy," the deliberate exposure to sunlight to treat various ailments, ranging from physical injuries to mental health conditions. Greeks believed that sunlight could purify the body, and they often constructed their homes and public spaces to maximize sunlight exposure, particularly for the ill.

In addition, Greek athletes were encouraged to exercise in the sun, believing that it would improve their physical condition and prepare them for competitions. Sunbathing, too, became a standard health practice used to strengthen the body and ward off disease.

The Romans: Public Health and the Sun

The Romans, known for their advancements in public health and architecture, also recognized the importance of sunlight for wellness. Roman baths, a central feature of their culture, were often designed with large windows to allow sunlight to flood the rooms, contributing to the overall sense of cleanliness, relaxation, and vitality. Romans believed that sunlight was essential for both physical strength and moral purity.

Roman physicians continued the tradition of heliotherapy, recommending sunlight exposure to cure various conditions, from skin diseases to respiratory ailments. Sunlight became intertwined with *balnea*, or therapeutic bathing, where sunlight and water were used to restore health.

Throughout these ancient civilizations, sunlight was more than just a natural element—it was a powerful symbol of health, healing, and life. These early insights laid the foundation for modern understandings of sunlight's essential role in human health, demonstrating that our ancestors recognized the profound connection between sunlight and well-being long before science could explain its mechanisms.

Sun Worship and Ancient Healing Practices

Across many ancient civilizations, sunlight was a source of physical nourishment and a symbol of divine power and spiritual healing. The sun was often regarded as a deity, revered for its life-giving energy, and its rays were believed to possess potent healing abilities. Sun worship and the belief in the sun's integral role in health and medicine formed a cornerstone of ancient cultures, shaping their medical practices, religious ceremonies, and daily rituals.

The Egyptians and Sun God Ra

In ancient Egypt, the sun was deeply tied to the divine through worshipping Ra, the sun god. Ra was considered the creator of all life, with his daily journey across the sky symbolizing the cycle of life, death, and rebirth. The Egyptians believed that sunlight carried Ra's life-giving energy, capable of rejuvenating both the body and the spirit.

The healing power of sunlight was also evident in their medicinal practices. Temples dedicated to Ra were often designed to maximize the sun's rays and were believed to purify and heal those who worshipped within. Priests and healers would prescribe sun exposure to the sick, especially those with skin conditions, assuming that sunlight could drive away illness and restore balance to the body. This connection between the divine sun and health reflected the Egyptians' holistic view of well-being, where spiritual and physical health were intertwined.

The Greeks and Heliotherapy

In ancient Greece, the sun was a symbol of health and a source of medical treatment. The Greeks revered Apollo, the god of the sun, light, and healing, thought to bring warmth and life to the world. In their view, sunlight was a pure, life-sustaining force that could prevent and cure illness.

Greek physicians, particularly Hippocrates, recognized sunlight's ability to enhance health. Hippocrates developed early forms of heliotherapy, which involved exposing patients to sunlight as a treatment for various conditions, including wounds, respiratory issues, and mental illness. The Greeks built sunrooms, or "solaria," where patients could bathe in the sun's healing rays.

Sunbathing was a practice for restoring physical health and fortifying mental clarity and emotional well-being, as sunlight was believed to bring harmony to the body and mind.

The Romans and Public Health

In Roman culture, sunlight was vital in public health and religious practice. The Romans worshipped Sol Invictus, the "Unconquered Sun," who was seen as a powerful, protective deity. Sol Invictus was often invoked in prayers for strength, protection, and healing. Sunlight was viewed as an agent of purification, and its warmth and brightness were believed to cleanse the body and spirit.

Romans incorporated sunlight into their health and architectural designs, constructing their famous public baths and spas with large, open windows to allow the sun's rays to enter. These spaces were considered both hygienic and therapeutic, combining the elements of water and sunlight to restore vitality. Roman physicians recommended regular exposure to sunlight to improve physical resilience, particularly for soldiers and athletes who needed to maintain peak conditions.

Sunlight as a Symbol of Purity and Vitality

For many ancient peoples, the sun's radiant light was synonymous with purity, health, and vitality. Sun worship extended beyond formal rituals into everyday life, influencing how people lived, worked, and healed. Sunlight was often invoked in purification ceremonies, believed to drive away evil spirits and illnesses. Its restorative power was thought to renew the body, cleanse the soul, and ensure prosperity.

The ancient understanding of sunlight as a divine, healing force was rooted in observation. People saw the difference in health between those who lived in sun-rich environments and those who did not. They recognized the sun's warmth as essential to agriculture, human energy, and healing. Though their explanations were spiritual, these early civilizations laid the groundwork for the modern understanding of sunlight's biological and psychological benefits.

In these ancient practices, we see the foundations of a belief that sunlight was more than just a physical force—a divine gift essential for spiritual and physical well-being. The reverence for the sun's healing powers helped shape early medical and religious practices, fostering a tradition that linked the sun's energy with life, health, and renewal.

Scientific Discovery of Sunlight's Benefits: From Heliotherapy to Modern Understanding of Sunlight's Biological Effects

As human societies evolved, the belief in the sun's healing powers, once rooted in spiritual practices, began to be explored through a scientific lens. From early forms of heliotherapy to modern medical research, scientists have uncovered numerous biological effects of sunlight, confirming its vital role in health. This chapter traces the journey from ancient sun-based treatments to the comprehensive understanding of sunlight's benefits we possess today.

Heliotherapy: The Birth of Sunlight Medicine

Heliotherapy—using sunlight to treat diseases—gained scientific recognition in the 19th century. "heliotherapy" comes from the Greek word *helios*, meaning "sun." Though early civilizations used the sun as a healing force, it wasn't until the 1800s that physicians formally studied its therapeutic properties.

One of the pioneers of heliotherapy was Danish physician Niels Ryberg Finsen, who developed light therapy to treat diseases such as lupus vulgaris (a form of skin tuberculosis). Finsen's groundbreaking work earned him the Nobel Prize in Medicine in 1903. He discovered that concentrated sunlight and artificial UV light could destroy bacteria, reduce inflammation, and stimulate the immune system. This early recognition of sunlight's antiseptic properties laid the foundation for further exploration of its benefits.

During the early 20th century, heliotherapy became widely popular, particularly in the treatment of tuberculosis, a leading cause of death at the time. Patients were prescribed controlled sun exposure at sanatoriums, designed with large outdoor areas to allow access to sunlight.

Physicians believed sunlight could help strengthen patients' lungs and immune systems, aiding their recovery from tuberculosis. This practice of heliotherapy eventually gave rise to modern phototherapy techniques.

The Discovery of Vitamin D and Rickets Prevention

One of the most significant scientific breakthroughs in understanding sunlight's health benefits was its role in producing vitamin D. In the early 20th century. Researchers identified that sunlight exposure helps the body synthesize vitamin D, which is crucial for bone health.

At that time, rickets—a disease that caused bone deformities in children—were widespread, particularly in urban areas where children had limited access to sunlight. Scientists realized that children who spent more time outdoors had more robust bones, leading them to investigate the link between sunlight and bone health. By the 1920s, researchers established that UV radiation from sunlight activates the production of vitamin D in the skin, which in turn helps the body absorb calcium and phosphorus, essential minerals for healthy bone development.

As a result of these findings, health campaigns in the 1930s and 1940s encouraged children to spend more time outside in the sun, and foods like milk were fortified with vitamin D to prevent rickets. This discovery marked a turning point in understanding how sunlight directly influences human health at a biochemical level.

Sunlight and Mental Health: The Role of Serotonin and Seasonal Affective Disorder (SAD)

In the 20th century, researchers began investigating the connection between sunlight and mental health, mainly how sunlight exposure affects mood. Studies revealed that sunlight stimulates the production of serotonin, a neurotransmitter that regulates mood, sleep, and feelings of well-being. Increased exposure to natural light during the day can boost serotonin levels, improving mood and mental clarity.

This discovery played a pivotal role in understanding Seasonal Affective Disorder (SAD), a form of depression that occurs during the winter months when sunlight exposure is limited. In the 1980s, Norman Rosenthal and his colleagues at the National Institute of Mental Health introduced the concept of SAD. They demonstrated that light therapy—exposure to bright artificial light—could effectively alleviate symptoms. Today, light therapy is a standard treatment for SAD, further affirming sunlight's impact on mental health.

Circadian Rhythms and Sleep Regulation

Another significant discovery was the relationship between sunlight and the body's circadian rhythms. Circadian rhythms are the body's internal clock, regulating sleep, alertness, and other biological functions over a 24-hour cycle. Sunlight, particularly in the morning, acts as a natural regulator of these rhythms by signaling to the brain that it's time to be awake and alert. This light exposure influences the production of melatonin, a hormone that controls sleep cycles.

Studies have shown that people exposed to natural sunlight in the morning have better sleep quality and are more alert during the day. Modern research has confirmed that disrupted exposure to natural light, such as spending too much time indoors or excessive use of artificial lighting at night, can lead to sleep disorders and negatively impact overall health. Understanding this connection has led to innovations in light therapy for improving sleep and adjusting to jet lag or shift work.

Sunlight's Role in Immune Function and Disease Prevention

The positive effects of sunlight on the immune system have become a key area of modern research. Sunlight exposure, particularly UVB rays, stimulates vitamin D production and directly influences immune cells. Vitamin D enhances the body's ability to fight off infections by promoting the activity of T-cells, which are essential in detecting and eliminating pathogens.

Researchers have also found that regular sunlight exposure reduces the risk of several chronic diseases, including cardiovascular diseases, certain types of cancer, and autoimmune disorders. A growing body of evidence suggests that people who live in regions with low sunlight exposure are more prone to developing these conditions, underscoring the importance of adequate sunlight for maintaining overall health.

Balancing Benefits and Risks: Sunlight and Skin Health

While the benefits of sunlight are well-documented, modern science has also highlighted the risks of overexposure, particularly the link between UV radiation and skin cancer. Prolonged exposure to UV rays can damage the skin's DNA, leading to premature aging and increasing the risk of skin cancer, including melanoma.

This dual understanding has led to a more nuanced approach to sunlight exposure: encouraging people to get enough sunlight for its health benefits while protecting their skin from overexposure through sunscreen, protective clothing, and moderation.

Conclusion: The Continuing Evolution of Sunlight Science

From its ancient roots in heliotherapy to modern discoveries in photo-biology, the scientific understanding of sunlight's role in human health has come a long way. Today, we know that sunlight plays a crucial role in physical health—through vitamin D production and immune function—and mental well-being and sleep regulation. Modern science continues to explore sunlight's vast potential to heal and protect while acknowledging the importance of managing exposure to balance its many benefits and risks.

Vitamin D – The Sunshine Vitamin

How Sunlight Stimulates Vitamin D Production: The Skin's Role in Synthesizing Vitamin D

Vitamin D is often called the "sunshine vitamin" because the body produces it when the skin is exposed to ultraviolet B (UVB) rays from sunlight. This process is essential for optimal health, as vitamin D is crucial in calcium absorption, bone health, immune function, and overall well-being. Here's an overview of how sunlight triggers vitamin D production in the skin:

The Process of Vitamin D Synthesis

UVB Rays and the Skin: When the skin is exposed to sunlight, specifically to UVB rays (which have wavelengths between 290 and 315 nanometers), these rays penetrate the outermost layer of the skin, called the **epidermis**. The UVB rays interact with a type of cholesterol found in the skin called **7-dehydrocholesterol**.

    Conversion to Pre-Vitamin D3: The UVB radiation converts

7-dehydrocholesterol into **previtamin D3** through **photochemical cleavage**. This is the first critical step in synthesizing vitamin D. This vitamin D3 is an inactive form that still needs further conversion to become biologically helpful.

Thermal Isomerization to Vitamin D3: Once pre-vitamin D3 is formed, it undergoes a natural thermal process in the skin called **isomerization**, which converts it into **cholecalciferol** (vitamin D3). This form of vitamin D3 is still inactive and needs to be activated by the liver and kidneys.

Activation of Vitamin D3: Vitamin D3 is released into the bloodstream from the skin and transported to the liver. In the liver, it is converted into **25-hydroxyvitamin D** (calcidiol), the primary circulating form of vitamin D. From the liver, calcidiol travels to the kidneys, where it is converted into **1,25-dihydroxyvitamin D** (calcitriol), the biologically active form of vitamin D.

The Role of Vitamin D in the Body

Once converted into its active form, calcitriol, vitamin D plays several critical roles in the body:

Calcium and Phosphate Absorption: Vitamin D helps the intestines absorb calcium and phosphate, minerals essential for bone health. This ensures strong bone formation, prevents bone diseases such as rickets in children and osteoporosis in adults, and supports muscle function.

Immune System Support: Vitamin D enhances the immune system by promoting the activity of T-cells, which are essential for defending the body against infections and diseases.

Regulation of Cell Growth: Vitamin D also regulates cell growth and differentiation, which is crucial for preventing certain types of cancer.

Factors Affecting Vitamin D Production

Several factors influence how efficiently the skin produces vitamin D, including:

Skin Type: People with lighter skin produce vitamin D more quickly because they have less melanin, which acts as a natural sunscreen. Those with darker skin require more sun exposure to produce the same amount of vitamin D.

Geographical Location: People who live closer to the equator receive more direct UVB rays throughout the year, leading to higher natural vitamin D production. Those living in northern or southern latitudes may struggle to get enough sunlight, especially during winter.

Time of Day: Vitamin D production is most efficient when the sun is high in the sky, typically between 10 a.m. and 3 p.m., as UVB rays are strongest during this period.

Age: As people age, their skin becomes less efficient at producing vitamin D. Older adults may require more sunlight or supplementation to maintain adequate levels.

Sunscreen and Clothing: While sunscreen is essential for preventing skin damage, it can also block UVB rays and limit vitamin D production. Similarly, clothing covering most of the skin reduces the area exposed to sunlight.

Balancing Sun Exposure and Health

While moderate sun exposure is essential for vitamin D production, it's crucial to balance it with skin protection to avoid overexposure, which can lead to skin damage and increase the risk of skin cancer. Many health experts recommend short periods of sun exposure—about 10 to 30 minutes, depending on skin type and location—several times a week to ensure sufficient vitamin D synthesis.

For individuals who cannot get enough sunlight due to geography, lifestyle, or health conditions, vitamin D can also be obtained through supplements and fortified foods. However, sunlight remains the most natural and influential source.

Sunlight is vital to the body's vitamin D production, demonstrating the connection between the environment and human health. Understanding how UVB rays activate this process allows us to appreciate sunlight's role in maintaining overall well-being.

Benefits of Vitamin D: Bone Health, Immune System Function, Mood Regulation

Vitamin D, often called the "sunshine vitamin," is crucial in many aspects of human health. It is produced in the skin when exposed to sunlight and can also be obtained from certain foods and supplements. This essential vitamin influences numerous bodily functions, and its deficiency can lead to various health problems. Below are the key benefits of vitamin D, focusing on bone health, immune system function, and mood regulation.

Bone Health: Supporting Strong Bones and Preventing Disease

Vitamin D is essential for the body to absorb calcium, which is necessary for building and maintaining strong bones. Without adequate vitamin D, the body cannot properly absorb calcium, weakening bones and various bone-related health issues.

Calcium Absorption: Vitamin D helps the intestines absorb calcium from the diet, ensuring enough calcium is available in the bloodstream to support bone mineralization.

Bone Growth and Maintenance: In children, vitamin D is crucial for proper bone development and preventing rickets, a condition characterized by soft, weak bones. In adults, vitamin D deficiency can lead to osteomalacia (softening of the bones) and osteoporosis, a condition where bones become brittle and prone to fractures.

Phosphorus Regulation: Along with calcium, vitamin D regulates phosphorus levels in the blood, another mineral essential for bone health and maintaining the strength of teeth.

Adequate vitamin D levels help ensure strong bone formation, reduce the risk of fractures in older adults, and promote overall skeletal health.

Immune System Function: Strengthening the Body's Defenses

Vitamin D is critical in regulating and enhancing the immune system, helping the body fight infections and diseases. Its role in immune health has been studied extensively, with significant evidence supporting its importance.

Activation of Immune Cells: Vitamin D enhances the pathogen-fighting effects of **monocytes** and **macrophages**—white blood cells that are part of the body's first line of defense. It also helps activate **T-cells**, which detect and eliminate pathogens such as bacteria and viruses.

Reducing the Risk of Infections: Studies have shown that people with adequate vitamin D levels are less likely to suffer from common illnesses, such as the flu, colds, and respiratory infections. Vitamin D may also help reduce the severity of infections when they do occur.

Autoimmune Disease Regulation: Vitamin D has anti-inflammatory properties, which can help regulate the immune response and prevent it from attacking the body's tissues. This makes it potentially beneficial in reducing the risk of autoimmune diseases such as multiple sclerosis, rheumatoid arthritis, and type 1 diabetes.

By strengthening the immune system, vitamin D enhances the body's ability to fend off illnesses and contributes to long-term immune health.

Mood Regulation: Improving Mental Health and Reducing Depression

One of vitamin D's lesser-known but increasingly studied benefits is its positive effect on mood and mental health. Sunlight, which helps the body produce vitamin D, has long been associated with improved mood, and research is uncovering the mechanisms behind this connection.

Serotonin Production: Vitamin D influences the production of **serotonin**, a neurotransmitter that significantly regulates mood. Higher levels of serotonin are linked to feelings of happiness and well-being, while lower levels are associated with depression and mood disorders.

Seasonal Affective Disorder (SAD): Vitamin D deficiency is often linked to **Seasonal Affective Disorder (SAD)**, a form of depression that occurs in the winter months when sunlight exposure is limited. Supplementing with vitamin D or using light therapy can help reduce symptoms of SAD, improving mood and energy levels.

Reducing the Risk of Depression: Several studies have suggested that low levels of vitamin D are associated with a higher risk of depression. Correcting vitamin D deficiency through supplements or increased sunlight exposure may help alleviate depressive symptoms, especially in those with clinically low levels of the vitamin.

By promoting serotonin production and regulating mood, vitamin D contributes to mental well-being and can help prevent and treat mood disorders such as depression and anxiety.

Conclusion: The Multifaceted Benefits of Vitamin D

Vitamin D plays a pivotal role in maintaining overall health, with its most notable benefits being:

Bone Health: Ensuring strong bones by enhancing calcium absorption and preventing bone-related diseases.

Immune System Function: Strengthening the body's defenses against infections and helping regulate immune responses.

Mood Regulation: Promoting mental well-being and reducing the risk of mood disorders, including depression and Seasonal Affective Disorder (SAD).

With such wide-ranging effects on health, it's essential to ensure that the body has adequate vitamin D levels, either through sensible sun exposure, diet, or supplementation.

Deficiency Risks and Modern Lifestyle Challenges: Why Many People Are Vitamin D Deficient Today

Despite the critical role that vitamin D plays in maintaining health, vitamin D deficiency has become a widespread issue, particularly in modern societies. The impact of modern lifestyles, technological advancements, and geographic conditions on this growing problem is significant. Below, we explore why many people are vitamin D deficient today and how modern lifestyles contribute to this issue, enlightening our understanding of this health concern.

Indoor Lifestyles: The Shift Away from Sunlight Exposure

One significant reason for widespread vitamin D deficiency is the modern shift toward indoor living. With advancements in technology and urbanization, many people now spend most of their time indoors at work, school, or home. This reduces opportunities for direct sunlight exposure, which is the body's primary source of vitamin D production.

Workplace and Leisure Habits: Most jobs today are office-based or involve indoor activities, keeping people out of the sun for long hours. Additionally, recreational activities, which once primarily took place outdoors, have shifted indoors, with people spending more time on computers, smartphones, and other devices.

Lack of Outdoor Time for Children: Children and adolescents also spend more time indoors, with reduced outdoor play and physical activity opportunities. This limits their exposure to sunlight during critical years for bone growth and development, increasing the risk of vitamin D deficiency from a young age.

The reliance on artificial lighting in modern homes and workplaces further exacerbates the issue, as indoor lighting does not provide the UVB rays necessary for vitamin D production.

Sunscreen Use: Balancing Protection and Vitamin D Production

While sunscreen is essential for protecting the skin from harmful UV radiation and preventing skin cancer, its widespread use has inadvertently contributed to vitamin D deficiency. Sunscreen works by blocking UVB rays, which are the same rays responsible for triggering vitamin D synthesis in the skin.

Sunscreen's Effectiveness: Sunscreens with a high sun protection factor (SPF), especially SPF 30 and above, can block up to 97% or more UVB rays. While this significantly reduces the risk of sunburn and skin cancer, it also dramatically decreases the skin's ability to produce vitamin D.

Widespread Use of Sunscreen: Health campaigns emphasizing sun safety have led to increased use of sunscreen, often applied in large amounts whenever people spend time outdoors. While this is critical for reducing the risk of sun damage, it also means that many individuals are not getting enough sunlight to produce adequate vitamin D, even outdoors.

To balance the need for sun protection with the benefits of vitamin D, experts often recommend getting short periods of sun exposure without sunscreen (around 10 to 30 minutes, depending on skin type) a few times a week.

Geographic Location: Limited Sunlight in Northern Latitudes

Geography significantly determines how much sunlight people receive throughout the year, especially in areas farther from the equator. In northern and southern latitudes, especially during the winter months, sunlight is much less intense, and UVB rays may not be strong enough to trigger vitamin D production in the skin.

Winter and Shorter Days: In regions with long winters, such as Northern Europe, Canada, and parts of the U.S., the shorter daylight hours and low sun angle result in minimal UVB exposure. This makes it difficult for people in these areas to produce enough vitamin D during winter, often leading to seasonal deficiencies.

High Latitudes: People living at high latitudes (above 37 degrees north or south) experience reduced UVB intensity year-round. As a result, they may need to rely more on dietary sources and supplements to maintain adequate vitamin D levels, especially in the absence of sufficient sunlight.

Cultural and Environmental Factors: In certain regions with extreme climates, like the Middle East, cultural practices may also limit sunlight exposure. For example, clothing that covers most of the skin for cultural or religious reasons can reduce the amount of sun reaching the skin, increasing the risk of vitamin D deficiency.

Aging and Skin's Decreased Ability to Synthesize Vitamin D

As people age, their skin becomes less efficient at synthesizing vitamin D. Older adults often have thinner skin and produce less

7-dehydrocholesterol, the precursor needed for the skin to generate vitamin D when exposed to UVB rays.

Higher Risk in Elderly Populations: This natural decrease in vitamin D production, combined with the fact that older adults may spend more time indoors, makes them particularly vulnerable to deficiency. Vitamin D deficiency in the elderly is linked to increased risks of osteoporosis, falls, fractures, and other health issues related to weakened bones and muscles.

Institutionalized or Homebound Individuals: Elderly individuals living in nursing homes or who are homebound are at an even greater risk, as they often receive minimal sunlight exposure. Vitamin D supplementation is often necessary for this group to maintain healthy levels.

Diet and Limited Vitamin D Sources

Unlike many other essential nutrients, vitamin D is not naturally abundant in many foods. The primary dietary sources of vitamin D include fatty fish (such as salmon, mackerel, and sardines), fortified foods (like milk, orange juice, and cereals), and egg yolks. However, many people do not consume these foods in sufficient quantities to meet their vitamin D needs through diet alone.

Lack of Dietary Intake: Obtaining enough vitamin D from food can be particularly challenging for people with dietary restrictions, such as vegetarians or vegans. Plant-based sources of vitamin D are limited, and fortified foods may not provide enough to meet daily requirements.

Reliance on Supplements: Given the limited dietary sources of vitamin D, many people need supplements to maintain adequate levels, mainly if they have limited sun exposure. However, not everyone knows their deficiency or the need for supplements, leading to widespread insufficiency.

Conclusion: Addressing Modern Vitamin D Deficiency

Modern lifestyles present significant challenges to maintaining adequate vitamin D levels, largely due to indoor living, sunscreen use, geographic limitations, and aging. While sun protection remains critical to prevent skin damage and cancer, balancing this with adequate sunlight exposure and possibly supplementing with vitamin D is necessary to prevent deficiency. Addressing this widespread issue requires greater awareness of vitamin D's importance and the factors contributing to its deficiency. By adopting balanced sun habits, considering dietary intake, and, when necessary, using supplements, individuals can take control of their health, mitigate the risks of vitamin D deficiency, and promote overall well-being.

3

Sunlight and Mental Well-Being

The Connection Between Sunlight and Serotonin: How Sunlight Boosts Serotonin and Affects Mood

Sunlight plays a vital role in regulating mood by boosting serotonin levels in the brain.

Serotonin is a neurotransmitter often referred to as the "feel-good" hormone because it contributes to feelings of well-being and happiness. The relationship between sunlight and serotonin is one of the reasons people often feel more energetic and positive during sunny days and more sluggish or down during darker months.

Sunlight and Serotonin Production

Exposure to sunlight stimulates the production of serotonin in the brain. Specifically, when sunlight hits the retina in the eyes, it triggers the release of serotonin through a pathway in the brain known as the hypothalamus. This process not only elevates mood but also enhances focus and calmness. Higher levels of serotonin help regulate mood, contributing to a greater sense of emotional balance.

Seasonal Affective Disorder (SAD)

A lack of sunlight, particularly in winter, can lead to lower serotonin levels. This decrease is often associated with **Seasonal Affective Disorder (SAD)**, a type of depression that occurs during seasons with less daylight. Individuals with SAD usually experience symptoms such as lethargy, mood swings, and low energy, all of which are linked to reduced serotonin levels.

Circadian Rhythm and Mood

Sunlight also affects the body's **circadian rhythm**, the internal clock that regulates sleep and wake cycles. Regular exposure to natural light helps maintain a healthy circadian rhythm, which supports mental health by promoting better sleep patterns and, subsequently, improved mood and energy levels.

Conclusion

In summary, sunlight significantly influences serotonin production, directly impacting mood and emotional well-being. Ensuring regular exposure to sunlight can help elevate serotonin levels, promote better sleep, and reduce the risk of mood disorders like depression, especially during seasons with shorter daylight hours.

Tackling Seasonal Affective Disorder (SAD): Understanding Reduced Sunlight and the Benefits of Light Therapy

Seasonal Affective Disorder (SAD) is a type of depression that occurs during certain seasons, most commonly in the winter months when there is reduced sunlight. SAD is linked to changes in the body's biological rhythms and a decrease in serotonin production, both of which contribute to mood disturbances. Understanding how reduced sunlight affects the brain and how light therapy can alleviate symptoms is critical to managing this condition.

How Reduced Sunlight Affects Mood

During winter, shorter days and longer nights reduce exposure to natural sunlight. This reduction in sunlight impacts the brain in several ways:

Lower Serotonin Levels: Sunlight is crucial for serotonin production, the neurotransmitter responsible for mood regulation. Less sunlight means less serotonin, which can lead to feelings of sadness, fatigue, and irritability.

Disrupted Circadian Rhythm: The body's internal clock, or **circadian rhythm**, relies on regular sunlight exposure to regulate sleep patterns. This rhythm can become misaligned with fewer daylight hours, leading to sleep disturbances and worsening mood symptoms.

Increased Melatonin Production: Less sunlight causes the brain to produce more **melatonin**, which induces sleep. Higher melatonin levels during the day can lead to fatigue and feelings of sluggishness, common symptoms of SAD.

Light Therapy as a Treatment for SAD

Light therapy, also known as phototherapy, is a standard and effective treatment for SAD. It involves using a special light box mimicking natural sunlight to compensate for the lack of exposure during winter. Here's how it works:

Boosting Serotonin: Exposure to bright light from a light box, usually in the morning, helps stimulate serotonin production, which can elevate mood and energy levels. Light therapy can gradually improve serotonin levels, counteracting the winter-induced drop.

Regulating Circadian Rhythm: Light therapy also helps to reset the circadian rhythm by signaling the brain that it is daytime. This helps regulate sleep-wake cycles, reduce daytime fatigue, and improve overall mood.

Reducing Melatonin Production: Therapy's bright light reduces melatonin production during the day, preventing the overwhelming feelings of tiredness and sluggishness associated with SAD.

Guidelines for Light Therapy

Light therapy should be used daily for effective treatment, ideally in the morning, for 20-30 minutes. The light box should emit around **10,000 lux**, a level that closely mimics outdoor sunlight. It is essential to consult a healthcare professional before beginning light therapy to ensure proper use and avoid side effects.

Conclusion

Reduced sunlight in winter can trigger Seasonal Affective Disorder by disrupting serotonin levels, circadian rhythms, and melatonin production. However, **light therapy** offers a practical and effective solution to combat these mood disturbances. By simulating natural sunlight, light therapy helps regulate mood, improve sleep, and restore energy levels, making it a valuable tool for those experiencing SAD.

The Role of Sunlight in Reducing Stress and Anxiety: Exploring the Calming Effects of Natural Light on Mental Health

Sunlight plays a vital role in maintaining not only physical health but also mental well-being. Numerous studies have shown that exposure to natural light can have a profound calming effect, reducing stress and anxiety levels. This is primarily due to sunlight's influence on key biological processes, such as serotonin production, circadian rhythm regulation, and vitamin D synthesis, all of which contribute to improved mood and reduced mental tension.

Sunlight Boosts Serotonin Levels

One of the most direct ways sunlight affects mental health is through its role in **serotonin production**. Serotonin is a neurotransmitter that contributes to happiness, calm, and emotional stability. When sunlight hits the retina, it signals the brain to release serotonin. This is why people often feel more positive, relaxed, and energized after spending time outdoors in the sun. Increased serotonin levels are closely linked to reduced anxiety and stress. When serotonin levels are low, people are more prone to feeling anxious or overwhelmed. By simply spending time in natural light, serotonin production can be enhanced, helping to alleviate symptoms of stress and anxiety.

Regulating the Circadian Rhythm

Sunlight also helps regulate the body's **circadian rhythm**, the internal clock that controls sleep-wake cycles. Regular exposure to natural light, especially in the morning, helps signal to the brain that it is daytime, promoting alertness and reducing feelings of lethargy or fogginess.

Proper circadian rhythm alignment contributes to better sleep, crucial for managing stress and anxiety. When individuals experience poor sleep or insomnia, stress hormones like **cortisol** can rise, exacerbating feelings of anxiety. Consistent exposure to sunlight helps ensure a healthy sleep-wake cycle, lowering stress levels and improving emotional resilience.

Sunlight and Vitamin D Synthesis

Exposure to sunlight enables the body to produce **vitamin D**, essential for brain health. Vitamin D has been shown to influence the production of mood-regulating neurotransmitters such as serotonin and dopamine. A deficiency in vitamin D is often associated with increased feelings of anxiety and depression.

In addition to its impact on mood, vitamin D reduces inflammation in the brain and supports nerve function, which is crucial for maintaining emotional balance. Regular sunlight exposure can help the body maintain adequate vitamin D levels, lowering anxiety and stress.

Nature and Sunlight: A Combined Effect

Spending time outdoors, particularly in natural settings, can amplify the stress-reducing effects of sunlight. Research shows that being in nature helps to lower **cortisol** levels, a hormone closely linked to stress. Sunlight, combined with the calming influence of nature, can promote relaxation, lower heart rate, and reduce anxiety symptoms.

The visual and sensory stimulation of natural environments and the physiological benefits of sunlight create a powerful combination that helps calm the mind and body. This is why activities like walking, hiking, or simply sitting in the sun can profoundly impact reducing stress.

Conclusion

Sunlight reduces stress and anxiety by boosting serotonin levels, regulating the circadian rhythm, and supporting vitamin D production.

Its calming effects can be further enhanced with time spent in nature. Regular exposure to sunlight improves mood and fosters long-term mental well-being by promoting relaxation and emotional balance. For those struggling with stress or anxiety, incorporating more time in natural light can be a simple yet effective strategy for improving mental health.

4

Circadian Rhythms and Sleep Regulation

How Sunlight Sets Your Internal Clock: The Relationship Between Morning Sunlight and Circadian Rhythm

Our bodies operate on a natural 24-hour cycle known as the **circadian rhythm**, which regulates many essential functions, including sleep, wakefulness, digestion, and hormone production.

Sunlight plays a crucial role in keeping this internal clock aligned with the external world, particularly in the morning. Understanding the relationship between morning sunlight and circadian rhythm can improve our sleep patterns, mental health, and overall well-being.

What is the Circadian Rhythm?

The **circadian rhythm** is the body's internal clock that governs the timing of physiological processes over a 24-hour cycle. It is regulated by the **suprachiasmatic nucleus (SCN)**, a group of cells in the brain's hypothalamus. This clock responds to exceptionally light environmental cues to stay synchronized with the Earth's day-night cycle.

The circadian rhythm controls vital functions such as:

Sleep and wake cycles: When we feel tired or alert.

Hormone production: Such as melatonin, which signals sleep, and cortisol, which promotes alertness.

Body temperature regulation and **metabolism**: Affecting energy levels throughout the day.

Morning Sunlight and Circadian Alignment

Morning sunlight has a powerful effect on regulating the circadian rhythm because of its influence on the **SCN**. When sunlight enters the eyes, light-sensitive cells in the retina send signals to the SCN, telling the brain that it is time to wake up and start the day. This process helps to align our internal clock with the external environment.

Melatonin Suppression: Morning sunlight halts melatonin production, the hormone responsible for inducing sleep. Melatonin levels typically rise in the evening, making us feel drowsy, and fall in the morning, as daylight signals the brain that it's time to be alert. Morning exposure to sunlight suppresses melatonin, making us feel more awake and energized.

Cortisol Release: Sunlight in the morning triggers the release of **cortisol**, a hormone that helps us feel alert and ready for the day. This natural rise in cortisol early in the day sets the stage for productivity and focus.

Setting the Sleep-Wake Cycle: By aligning our circadian rhythm with sunlight's natural rise and fall, our bodies learn when to feel sleepy and when to wake up. Regular exposure to morning sunlight helps solidify this rhythm, improving the quality and consistency of sleep.

The Importance of Blue Light in the Morning

Morning sunlight is rich in **blue light**, a particularly effective wavelength in regulating the circadian rhythm. Blue light has the most substantial impact on the SCN, making morning sunlight the ideal cue to reset the body's internal clock daily. Exposure to blue light early in the morning is essential for reinforcing the wake-up signal and maintaining a healthy sleep-wake cycle.

Conversely, exposure to blue light from artificial sources (such as screens) late at night can disrupt the circadian rhythm by delaying the release of melatonin, leading to poor sleep quality. This is why it's recommended to minimize screen time before bed and seek out natural sunlight in the morning to set the internal clock properly.

Benefits of Morning Sunlight for Mental and Physical Health

By synchronizing the circadian rhythm with morning sunlight, individuals can experience significant benefits for both mental and physical health:

Improved Sleep: A well-regulated circadian rhythm promotes more restful and restorative sleep. People who consistently get morning sunlight tend to fall asleep more easily, stay asleep longer, and feel refreshed.

Boosted Mood and Energy: Sunlight exposure helps increase serotonin production, which improves mood and energy levels throughout the day. This is particularly important for people who struggle with mood disorders like **Seasonal Affective Disorder (SAD)** during months with limited sunlight.

Enhanced Focus and Productivity: Morning sunlight helps regulate the body's production of cortisol and other hormones associated with alertness and concentration, leading to improved productivity and cognitive function during the day.

Strategies to Maximize Morning Sunlight Exposure

To harness the benefits of morning sunlight and regulate the circadian rhythm, consider the following strategies:

Spend time outside: Aim to spend at least 15–30 minutes outdoors in the morning sunlight. Even on cloudy days, natural light is beneficial.

Keep blinds open: Allow sunlight to enter your home in the morning by keeping curtains or blinds open, particularly in the bedroom.

Avoid sunglasses early in the day: While sunglasses are essential for eye protection, try to avoid them during early morning exposure to maximize light absorption through your eyes.

Take a morning walk: A walk outside in the morning provides sunlight exposure and encourages physical activity, further enhancing energy and mood.

Conclusion

Morning sunlight is essential for maintaining a healthy circadian rhythm, affecting our sleep, mood, and overall health. By aligning our internal clock with the natural rise and fall of the sun, we can improve our energy levels, sleep quality, and mental well-being. Incorporating more exposure to natural light, particularly in the morning, is a simple but powerful way to regulate our biological clock and enhance our daily lives.

The Importance of Morning Exposure to Sunlight: How Early Sunlight Improves Sleep Quality

Morning exposure to sunlight is one of the simplest and most effective ways to improve sleep quality. This natural light helps regulate the body's internal clock, known as the **circadian rhythm**. It influences the production of critical hormones like **melatonin** and **cortisol** that directly affect sleep and wakefulness. We can optimize our sleep patterns by aligning our internal rhythms with natural daylight cycles, leading to better overall health and well-being.

Regulating the Circadian Rhythm

The **circadian rhythm** is the body's internal 24-hour clock that regulates sleep, wakefulness, and other biological processes. Exposure to natural light, especially in the morning, helps synchronize this internal clock with the external environment. Morning sunlight provides a powerful signal to the brain that it's time to be awake and alert, helping to set the daily rhythm. When the circadian rhythm is aligned correctly, melatonin production occurs at the right time—usually in the evening—making it easier to fall asleep and stay asleep. Regular morning sunlight exposure can prevent the misalignment of this rhythm, which often leads to insomnia, difficulty waking up, or poor sleep quality.

Suppressing Melatonin in the Morning

Melatonin is the hormone that signals the body it's time to sleep. Its production naturally increases in the evening as light levels decrease, promoting sleepiness. However, sunlight exposure signals the brain to stop melatonin production in the morning. This suppression of melatonin helps us feel more awake and alert during the day.

Without sufficient exposure to morning light, melatonin production may linger into the daytime, making us dizzy and affecting our energy levels. By resetting melatonin production early in the day with sunlight, the body can better regulate its sleep-wake cycle, leading to more restful sleep at night.

Stimulating Cortisol Production

Cortisol, often known as the "stress hormone," is released at higher levels in the morning and helps promote alertness and energy for the day ahead. Morning sunlight triggers the production of cortisol at the right time, helping to wake us up naturally and stay focused throughout the day. This process is known as the **cortisol awakening response (CAR)**.

A well-timed cortisol boost in the morning improves mood, productivity, and overall alertness. It also ensures that cortisol levels decline later in the day, making it easier for the body to transition into a relaxed state before bedtime, enhancing sleep quality.

Blue Light in the Morning vs. Artificial Blue Light at Night

Sunlight in the morning contains higher amounts of **blue light**, which is particularly effective at regulating the circadian rhythm. This blue light helps the brain recognize daytime and resets the internal clock accordingly. Getting blue light exposure early in the day is essential for maintaining a healthy sleep-wake cycle.

However, exposure to blue light from artificial sources, such as smartphones or computer screens, can disrupt this process late at night. Blue light in the evening can delay the release of melatonin, making it harder to fall asleep. This is why getting sunlight in the morning and minimizing artificial blue light exposure before bed is essential.

Improved Sleep Quality and Duration

By aligning the body's circadian rhythm with natural sunlight, individuals can experience: **Easier time falling asleep:** Proper morning sunlight exposure helps the body naturally produce melatonin at night, making it easier to fall asleep at an appropriate time.

Better sleep duration: A well-regulated circadian rhythm reduces nighttime awakenings and promotes more profound, restorative sleep.

More consistent sleep patterns: Exposure to morning sunlight reinforces a regular sleep schedule, reducing the likelihood of insomnia or erratic sleep patterns.

Practical Ways to Increase Morning Sunlight Exposure

To harness the benefits of morning sunlight and improve sleep quality, here are some practical tips:

Spend at least 15-30 minutes outside in the morning: Aim to get direct sunlight exposure as early as possible.

Open your blinds or curtains: Allow natural sunlight to flood your home or workspace in the morning.

Exercise outdoors: A morning walk or outdoor workout can combine the benefits of physical activity and unlight exposure, boosting mood and energy levels.

Avoid sunglasses early in the morning: While sunglasses are essential for eye protection, try to avoid wearing them briefly during sunlight to maximize light absorption.

Conclusion

Morning exposure to sunlight is essential for regulating the circadian rhythm and improving sleep quality. By stimulating melatonin suppression and cortisol production and aligning the body's internal clock, sunlight helps us feel awake and energized during the day and sleep soundly at night. Incorporating more morning sunlight into your routine can lead to more restful sleep, better mood, and enhanced overall well-being.

Overcoming Sleep Disorders with Light Therapy: How Light Exposure Can Combat Insomnia and Other Sleep-Related Issues

Light therapy is a proven and effective treatment for various sleep disorders, particularly those that involve disruptions to the body's internal clock, known as the **circadian rhythm**. By carefully timed exposure to bright light, individuals can adjust their sleep-wake cycles, reduce insomnia symptoms, and improve overall sleep quality. Light therapy is beneficial in addressing conditions like **insomnia**, **Delayed Sleep Phase Syndrome (DSPS)**, and **Seasonal Affective Disorder (SAD)**, all of which are linked to irregular or insufficient exposure to natural light.

The Role of Light in Regulating Sleep

Our circadian rhythm, a 24-hour internal clock that controls sleep-wake cycles, is heavily influenced by light, particularly natural sunlight. Exposure to light, especially in the morning, sends signals to the brain, helping to regulate hormones like **melatonin** (which promotes sleep) and **cortisol** (which helps with wakefulness). When light exposure is inconsistent or insufficient, it can disrupt the circadian rhythm, leading to various sleep problems.

Light therapy involves using a lightbox that mimics natural sunlight to reset the circadian rhythm and address sleep-related issues. By providing the brain with the right light signals at the correct times of day, light therapy helps recalibrate the body's internal clock and promote better sleep patterns.

Light Therapy for Insomnia

Insomnia is one of the most common sleep disorders and is characterized by difficulty falling asleep, staying asleep, or waking up too early.

One of the underlying causes of insomnia can be a misaligned circadian rhythm. This is where light therapy can help, by using exposure to bright light at specific times of the day to reset the sleep-wake cycle.

Morning Light Exposure: For those with **delayed sleep onset** (difficulty falling asleep at night), light therapy in the morning helps advance the circadian rhythm, making it easier to fall asleep earlier in the evening and wake up on time in the morning.

Evening Light Exposure: For those with **advanced sleep phase syndrome** (feeling sleepy too early in the evening), light therapy later in the day can delay the internal clock, helping individuals stay awake longer and sleep later.

Light therapy can help those suffering from insomnia achieve more consistent and restful sleep by resetting the circadian rhythm.

Light Therapy for Delayed Sleep Phase Syndrome (DSPS)

Delayed Sleep Phase Syndrome (DSPS) is when a person's internal clock is shifted later than the typical sleep-wake schedule, leading them to fall asleep and wake up much later than desired. This misalignment can cause significant disruptions to daily life, particularly for students or working professionals.

For individuals with DSPS, **morning light therapy** is a crucial treatment. Exposure to bright light in the early morning hours helps shift the circadian rhythm earlier, encouraging the body to fall asleep and wake up at more conventional times. Over time, this can help people with DSPS align their sleep patterns with societal norms and improve their overall functioning.

Light Therapy for Seasonal Affective Disorder (SAD)

Seasonal Affective Disorder (SAD) is a type of depression that occurs during the fall and winter months when there is less natural sunlight.

SAD is closely linked to circadian rhythm disruptions and a reduction in serotonin levels, which can also affect sleep patterns. Many people with SAD experience **insomnia**, excessive sleepiness, or a disrupted sleep-wake cycle. Light therapy, particularly with a **10,000-lux lightbox**, can effectively treat both the mood and sleep-related symptoms of SAD. By mimicking natural sunlight, light therapy helps regulate melatonin and serotonin production, leading to better mood regulation and improved sleep.

Regular exposure to bright light in the morning helps those with SAD maintain a more balanced circadian rhythm, improving mood and sleep quality during the darker months.

How Light Therapy Works

Light therapy involves sitting in front of a lightbox that emits bright light, usually at **10,000 lux**—a much higher intensity than regular indoor lighting. The light is typically white or blue-toned, mimicking the effect of natural daylight. A typical session lasts about **20–30 minutes** and is most effective when done in the morning. Consistency is vital, as daily exposure to light is necessary to help the body reset its internal clock.

The therapy's bright light signals the brain that it is daytime, reducing melatonin production and boosting alertness. Over time, this helps re-align the circadian rhythm, promoting more restful sleep at night and reducing the risk of sleep disturbances.

Benefits of Light Therapy for Sleep Disorders

Light therapy is a drug-free and natural treatment that leverages the body's natural response to light.

Improved sleep quality: By resetting the circadian rhythm, light therapy helps reduce nighttime awakenings, improve sleep onset, and enhance overall sleep quality.

Boosted mood and energy: Since light therapy also increases serotonin levels and helps regulate cortisol, it can improve energy and mood, especially for those with SAD.

Safety and Precautions

While light therapy is generally safe, proper guidelines must be followed to avoid potential side effects such as headaches, eye strain, or nausea. Individuals with certain medical conditions, such as bipolar disorder or light sensitivity, should consult a healthcare provider before starting light therapy. It is also essential to use light therapy at the correct time of day; too late can delay the circadian rhythm and make it harder to fall asleep at night.

Conclusion

Light therapy is a practical, natural solution for managing sleep disorders like insomnia, Delayed Sleep Phase Syndrome, and Seasonal Affective Disorder. By controlled exposure to bright light, individuals can reset their circadian rhythm, improve sleep quality, and experience better overall well-being. Light therapy offers a simple yet powerful tool for those who struggle with sleep-related issues to regain control of their sleep-wake cycle and enjoy more restful, rejuvenating sleep.

5

Sunlight and Skin Health

Sunlight as Therapy for Skin Conditions: How Moderate UV Exposure Benefits Psoriasis, Eczema, and Acne

While excessive exposure to ultraviolet (UV) light from the sun can be harmful, **moderate UV exposure** can offer therapeutic benefits for specific skin conditions, including **psoriasis, eczema,** and **acne.** The controlled use of sunlight, often called **phototherapy,** has been a long-standing treatment option for individuals with chronic skin conditions. In this context, sunlight, particularly **UVB rays,** can help reduce inflammation, slow the rapid skin cell turnover associated with these conditions, and alleviate symptoms.

Sunlight and Psoriasis

Psoriasis is a chronic autoimmune condition characterized by the rapid growth of skin cells, leading to thick, scaly patches of skin that are often itchy and painful. Moderate exposure to sunlight, specifically

UVB rays, has been shown to help slow down excessive skin cell production and reduce the symptoms of psoriasis.

How UV Exposure Helps: UVB light penetrates the skin and helps reduce the abnormal activity of the immune system, which is responsible for the overproduction of skin cells. This leads to thinner, smoother skin and less severe psoriatic lesions.

Phototherapy for Psoriasis: In clinical settings, **narrowband UVB phototherapy** treats moderate to severe psoriasis. This therapy mimics the beneficial effects of sunlight, allowing individuals to experience the therapeutic benefits of UV exposure in a controlled environment, reducing the risk of overexposure.

Moderate sunlight exposure can also help improve **psoriasis-related symptoms** in individuals who may not have access to professional phototherapy. However, overexposure should be avoided, as it can trigger a flare-up or increase the risk of skin damage.

Sunlight and Eczema

Eczema, or **atopic dermatitis**, is a common inflammatory skin condition that causes itchy, red, and inflamed patches of skin. Sunlight, and particularly UVB rays, can also be beneficial in treating eczema by reducing inflammation and soothing irritated skin.

Reducing Inflammation: Moderate exposure to UVB light helps reduce the inflammation associated with eczema, making the skin less red and irritated. The light suppresses the immune response in the skin, which leads to flare-ups and itchy rashes typical of eczema.

Improving Skin Barrier Function: Sunlight can also promote the production of **vitamin D**, which improves skin barrier function. A healthier skin barrier helps protect against irritants and allergens, reducing the likelihood of eczema flare-ups.

As with psoriasis, **narrowband UVB phototherapy** is also used to treat severe eczema. This controlled exposure helps reduce the severity of symptoms without the side effects associated with long-term steroid use.

Sunlight and Acne

Acne is a common skin condition caused by clogged pores, bacteria, and inflammation. Although sunlight alone cannot completely cure acne, moderate UV exposure can help reduce the appearance of acne by controlling bacterial growth and reducing inflammation.

Bacterial Reduction: UV light has mild antibacterial properties, which can help kill the bacteria that contribute to acne formation. By reducing the bacterial load on the skin, UV exposure can help lessen the severity of acne breakouts.

Reduction in Inflammation: UV light can also help reduce the inflammation associated with acne, leading to fewer red and swollen pimples. This effect can make acne appear less severe and lead to faster healing of existing lesions.

However, excessive sun exposure can worsen acne by causing the skin to produce more oil or increasing irritation. Therefore, any sunlight therapy for acne must be approached with caution to avoid long-term damage.

Benefits of Moderate Sunlight Exposure

Moderate exposure to sunlight offers several benefits for skin conditions like psoriasis, eczema, and acne:

Slows Skin Cell Turnover: For psoriasis, UVB light slows down the rapid skin cell production that causes scaly patches, leading to smoother, clearer skin.

Reduces Inflammation: UV light helps reduce the inflammation that triggers flare-ups and breakouts in eczema and acne, providing relief from symptoms.

Antibacterial Properties: UV light helps reduce acne-causing bacteria on the skin's surface, helping to clear blemishes.

Promotes Vitamin D Production: Sunlight stimulates the skin to produce **vitamin D**, a nutrient essential for healthy skin function. Vitamin D has been shown to regulate the immune response in the skin, which can help manage conditions like eczema.

Cautions and Considerations

While sunlight can provide therapeutic benefits, practicing moderation and avoiding overexposure is essential. Too much UV light can increase the risk of skin damage, sunburn, and long-term issues like premature aging and skin cancer.

Sunscreen Use: If you plan to spend extended periods in the sun, applying a **broad-spectrum sunscreen** to protect against UVA and excessive UVB rays is essential. Sunscreen should be applied to unaffected areas of skin to prevent sun damage while allowing limited exposure to areas affected by skin conditions.

Professional Guidance: Individuals with severe skin conditions should consult with a dermatologist or healthcare provider before using sunlight as a therapy. In many cases, **narrowband UVB phototherapy** in a clinical setting may provide a safer and more controlled treatment option.

Conclusion

Moderate exposure to sunlight, particularly UVB rays, offers therapeutic benefits for individuals suffering from psoriasis, eczema, and acne. Sunlight can help slow down the rapid skin cell turnover in psoriasis, reduce inflammation in eczema, and control bacterial growth and inflammation in acne. However, it is crucial to balance the benefits of sunlight with the potential risks of overexposure. It is essential to consult with a healthcare professional for guidance on appropriate light exposure or phototherapy treatments. By incorporating moderate sunlight into their skincare regimen, individuals with these skin conditions may experience improved symptoms and a better quality of life.

Understand Phototherapy, which is the therapeutic use of UV light in treating various skin disorders.

Phototherapy is a medical treatment that uses controlled exposure to **ultraviolet (UV) light** to treat various skin disorders. It is particularly effective for conditions like **psoriasis, eczema,** and **vitiligo**, and in some cases, it can be beneficial for **acne** and **Seasonal Affective Disorder (SAD).**

There are different types of UV light used in phototherapy, but the two most common types are:

UVB Light (Ultraviolet B):

Narrowband UVB therapy is the most widely used and is effective in treating psoriasis, eczema, and vitiligo. It slows down abnormal skin cell growth, reduces inflammation, and helps relieve symptoms.

Broadband UVB therapy is an older form but is still used in some instances. It is slightly less targeted than narrowband UVB therapy.

PUVA Therapy (Psoralen + UVA):

This therapy involves taking **psoralen**, which makes the skin more sensitive to UVA light. It's used for more severe skin conditions like psoriasis and vitiligo.

Phototherapy sessions are usually conducted in a healthcare setting under the supervision of a dermatologist, ensuring the UV light is delivered safely and at the correct dosage to prevent side effects such as burning or skin damage.

While phototherapy is a powerful tool for managing skin conditions, it is essential to consult a healthcare provider to determine the appropriate type and duration of treatment. Proper monitoring ensures that you gain the benefits of UV light without the risks associated with excessive exposure.

Balancing Skin Health and Protection: The Need for Safe Sun Exposure and the Risks of Overexposure

Sunlight offers a range of health benefits, including **vitamin D production**, improved **mood**, and therapeutic effects on skin conditions like **psoriasis** and **eczema**. However, achieving these benefits requires a careful balance between getting enough sun and avoiding the risks of **overexposure**, such as **sunburn** and **skin cancer**. Understanding how to enjoy safe sun exposure while minimizing risks is crucial for maintaining overall skin health.

Benefits of Safe Sun Exposure

Moderate and safe exposure to sunlight has numerous benefits for both physical and mental well-being:

Vitamin D Production: Sunlight stimulates the production of **vitamin D**, which is essential for bone health, immune function, and mood regulation. A lack of vitamin D can lead to deficiencies that cause weakened bones (e.g., rickets or osteoporosis) and other health problems.

Mood Enhancement: Sunlight boosts the production of **serotonin**, a neurotransmitter associated with happiness and calmness. Regular sun exposure, especially in the morning, can help improve mood and reduce symptoms of **Seasonal Affective Disorder (SAD)** and mild depression.

Skin Therapy: Moderate exposure to UV light can help treat skin conditions like **psoriasis**, **eczema**, and **acne** by reducing inflammation, slowing down excessive skin cell growth, and improving symptoms.

The Risks of Overexposure

While sunlight is beneficial, **overexposure to UV radiation**—both **UVA** and **UVB rays**—can cause severe damage to the skin. Understanding these risks is essential for protecting yourself:

Sunburn: Overexposure to the sun, especially without proper protection, can lead to **sunburn**, which causes the skin to become red, painful, and inflamed. Sunburn is an immediate sign of skin damage and increases the risk of further complications, including long-term skin damage.

Skin Aging (Photoaging): Prolonged exposure to UV rays accelerates skin aging, a process called **photoaging**. This leads to **wrinkles**, **sunspots**, **loss of skin elasticity**, and a leathery texture.

Skin Cancer: The most severe consequence of overexposure to UV radiation is the increased risk of developing **skin cancer**, including **basal cell carcinoma**, **squamous cell carcinoma**, and **melanoma**. UV radiation can damage the DNA in skin cells, leading to mutations that trigger cancer development.

Melanoma, the most dangerous form of skin cancer, is mainly linked to episodes of severe sunburn and cumulative UV exposure over time. Protecting your skin from overexposure can significantly reduce the risk of developing skin cancer.

Strategies for Safe Sun Exposure

To strike the right balance between gaining the benefits of sunlight and avoiding its harmful effects, it's essential to follow these strategies:

Limit Exposure During Peak Hours: UV rays are strongest between **10 a.m. and 4 p.m.**, so limit sun exposure. If you need to be outside, seek shade, wear protective clothing, or use Sunscreen.

Use Sunscreen Regularly: Apply a **broad-spectrum sunscreen** with at least **SPF 30** to protect against UVA and UVB rays. Reapply every two hours, especially after swimming or sweating.

Wear Protective Clothing: Long-sleeved shirts, wide-brimmed hats, and sunglasses can provide additional protection outdoors. Specialized UV-blocking clothing is also available to defend against the sun's harmful rays.

Gradual Sun Exposure: If you are not used to being in the sun, build up exposure gradually to allow your skin to adjust without getting burned.

Monitor UV Index: The **UV index** measures the sun's intensity on a given day. A higher UV index means a greater risk of skin damage, so it's essential to take extra precautions when the index is high.

Avoid Tanning Beds: Tanning beds emit concentrated UV radiation that significantly increases the risk of skin cancer. It's safer to achieve a tan gradually through limited natural sun exposure or use sunless tanning products as a safer alternative.

Special Considerations for Skin Conditions

Sunlight can offer therapeutic benefits for individuals with skin conditions like **psoriasis** or **eczema**, but overexposure can still pose risks. Controlled **phototherapy** under medical supervision is often recommended to ensure the right balance of UV exposure, minimizing the risk of damage while providing therapeutic benefits.

Additionally, some individuals with skin conditions may be more sensitive to UV radiation, so it is crucial to work closely with a dermatologist to manage sun exposure.

Conclusion

Balancing skin health and sun protection involves getting enough sunlight to reap its benefits—like vitamin D production and improved mood—while avoiding overexposure that leads to sunburn, premature aging, and skin cancer. Strategies such as wearing Sunscreen, limiting exposure during peak hours, and gradually increasing time in the sun can help you safely enjoy the advantages of sunlight while minimizing the risks. This balance is critical to maintaining healthy, vibrant skin while protecting against the long-term dangers of UV radiation.

6

Boosting the Immune System with Sunlight

The Role of Sunlight in Immune Function: How Sunlight Activates T-Cells and Strengthens the Immune Response

Sunlight is crucial in supporting and strengthening the immune system, primarily through its effects on the body's **T-cells**—a type of white blood cell essential for immune defense. T-cells are responsible for identifying and attacking foreign pathogens like viruses and bacteria.

Research has shown that **moderate sunlight exposure** can help activate these cells and improve overall immune function.

How Sunlight Activates T-Cells

One key way sunlight boosts the immune system is through its impact on **vitamin D production**. When the skin is exposed to **UVB rays** from sunlight, it triggers the production of **vitamin D**. This vitamin is vital for various immune functions, including the activation of **T-cells**.

Vitamin D and T-Cell Activation: When vitamin D is present in the body, it helps T-cells transition from a dormant state to an active one, enabling them to respond to pathogens more effectively. Without sufficient vitamin D, T-cells remain inactive and less capable of fighting off infections.

Direct Sunlight and T-Cell Mobility: Recent studies suggest that sunlight may also have a more direct impact on the immune system, aside from vitamin D. A study published in *Scientific Reports* found that **blue light** from sunlight can increase the motility of T-cells, making them more active and efficient in their function. This suggests that sunlight directly enhances the ability of T-cells to move through the body and respond to infections more quickly.

Strengthening the Immune Response

By activating T-cells, sunlight helps improve the body's ability to identify and eliminate harmful pathogens. With adequate sunlight exposure, the immune system becomes more responsive, better equipped to fend off infections, and more efficient at controlling inflammation.

Immune Regulation: Vitamin D, produced through sunlight exposure, also regulates the immune system. It helps modulate the immune response, preventing it from overreacting and reducing the risk of autoimmune conditions, where the immune system mistakenly attacks healthy tissues.

Reducing Inflammation: Sunlight helps regulate immune function by controlling **inflammation**, the body's natural response to infection or injury. Chronic inflammation, if left unchecked, can lead to various diseases. Vitamin D's anti-inflammatory properties help keep inflammation healthy, protecting tissues from damage.

The Impact of Vitamin D Deficiency

Inadequate sunlight exposure, particularly in areas with long winters or limited sunlight, can lead to **vitamin D deficiency**, compromising immune function. People with vitamin D deficiency are more susceptible to **the common cold**, flu, and other respiratory infections.

Weakened Immune Defense: Without enough vitamin D, the immune system struggles to activate T-cells effectively, leading to a slower response to infections. This leaves the body more vulnerable to illness and less capable of managing inflammatory responses.

Increased Autoimmune Risk: Studies have also linked vitamin D deficiency to an increased risk of developing autoimmune diseases, such as **multiple sclerosis, rheumatoid arthritis**, and **type 1 diabetes**, where the immune system mistakenly attacks the body's tissues.

Optimal Sunlight Exposure for Immune Health

Moderate sun exposure is critical to maximizing the immune-boosting benefits of sunlight. Here are some guidelines for safe and effective sunlight exposure:

Timing: Spending **10 to 30 minutes** in direct sunlight several times a week can help the body produce enough vitamin D. The exact amount of time varies depending on skin type, location, and the time of year.

Areas of Exposure: Exposing larger areas of the skin, such as the arms, legs, or back, is more effective at generating vitamin D than exposing smaller areas like the hands or face.

Sunscreen and Balance: While sunlight is essential for vitamin D production, overexposure can increase the risk of skin damage and skin cancer. It's critical to find a balance between gaining enough sun exposure for immune health while protecting the skin from overexposure by wearing sunscreen or covering up after the recommended time in the sun.

Sunlight and Immune Function During Winter

During the winter months, many people experience reduced exposure to sunlight, which can lead to a drop in vitamin D levels. This seasonal dip in sunlight often correlates with increased illnesses like colds and the flu. To maintain immune function during the winter, some individuals may benefit from **vitamin D supplementation** or other sources of vitamin D, such as fortified foods and fatty fish.

Conclusion

Sunlight plays a crucial role in immune function by activating T-cells and facilitating vitamin D production, a key player in immune regulation. Regular, moderate sunlight exposure helps the immune system respond effectively to infections while controlling inflammation. However, balancing adequate sun exposure and skin protection is essential for maintaining immune health and overall well-being. For those living in areas with limited sunlight, especially in the winter, maintaining optimal vitamin D levels through supplements or diet is essential for sustaining a healthy immune system.

Sunlight, Autoimmune Disorders, and Inflammation: Exploring the Relationship Between Sunlight, Vitamin D, and Reduced Inflammation in Autoimmune Conditions

The relationship between **sunlight**, **vitamin D**, and the immune system is vital for understanding how exposure to sunlight can affect autoimmune disorders and inflammation. Autoimmune diseases occur when the body's immune system mistakenly attacks its tissues, leading to chronic inflammation and tissue damage. Adequate exposure to sunlight, which stimulates vitamin D production, is crucial in modulating immune function and reducing inflammation in individuals with autoimmune disorders.

Sunlight and Vitamin D Production

When skin is exposed to **ultraviolet B (UVB)** rays from sunlight, it triggers the production of **vitamin D** in the body. This vitamin is crucial for regulating immune function and maintaining the balance between pro-inflammatory and anti-inflammatory responses in the immune system.

Vitamin D is essential for activating and controlling **T-cells**, the immune cells that play a central role in defending the body against infections. It also has an anti-inflammatory effect, which is significant in managing autoimmune diseases where inflammation is a hallmark symptom. Without sufficient vitamin D, the immune system can become dysregulated, leading to an increased risk of autoimmune conditions and chronic inflammation.

The Link Between Vitamin D Deficiency and Autoimmune Diseases

Research has shown that **vitamin D deficiency** is associated with an increased risk of developing autoimmune diseases, including **multiple sclerosis (MS)**, **rheumatoid arthritis (RA)**, **systemic lupus erythematosus (SLE)**, and **type 1 diabetes**. The immune system mistakenly attacks healthy cells in these conditions, causing inflammation and tissue damage.

Multiple Sclerosis (MS): MS is a disease in which the immune system attacks the protective covering of nerve fibers in the central nervous system. Studies have shown that individuals living in regions with low sunlight exposure are at a higher risk of developing MS, and vitamin D levels are inversely correlated with disease activity. Adequate sunlight exposure and vitamin D supplementation have reduced the risk of MS onset and progression.

Rheumatoid Arthritis (RA): RA is an autoimmune condition where the immune system attacks the joints, leading to chronic inflammation and pain. Vitamin D has been shown to suppress the overactive immune responses in RA, helping to reduce inflammation and improve symptoms.

Low vitamin D levels are expected in individuals with RA and are linked to more severe disease activity.

Systemic Lupus Erythematosus (SLE): In SLE, the immune system attacks various organs and tissues, leading to widespread inflammation. While individuals with SLE are often advised to avoid excessive sun exposure due to photosensitivity, maintaining adequate vitamin D levels is crucial for controlling immune responses and reducing inflammation in this condition.

Sunlight's Role in Reducing Inflammation

Vitamin D produced through sunlight exposure has potent **anti-inflammatory properties**. In autoimmune conditions, inflammation is a primary cause of tissue damage, and reducing this inflammation is critical to managing symptoms. Here's how sunlight and vitamin D help reduce inflammation:

Modulating T-Cell Activity: Vitamin D plays a regulatory role in **T-cell function**. It helps balance **pro-inflammatory T-helper cells (Th1 and Th17)** and **anti-inflammatory regulatory T-cells (Tregs)**. This balance is often disrupted in autoimmune disorders, leading to an overactive immune response and excessive inflammation. Vitamin D helps restore this balance by promoting the activity of Tregs, which suppress the inflammatory immune response.

Inhibiting Cytokine Production: Inflammation is driven by **cytokine** signaling molecules that promote immune activity. In autoimmune diseases, the immune system produces excessive pro-inflammatory cytokines, perpetuating the inflammation cycle. Vitamin D helps reduce the production of these cytokines, particularly **interleukin-6 (IL-6)** and **tumor necrosis factor-alpha (TNF-alpha)**, both of which play significant roles in chronic inflammation.

Regulating Immune Responses: Sunlight stimulates vitamin D production And helps regulate immune responses by preventing excessive or prolonged inflammation. This is particularly beneficial for individuals with autoimmune disorders, where the immune system must be carefully modulated to avoid tissue damage.

Managing Autoimmune Disorders Through Safe Sunlight Exposure

While sunlight is beneficial for increasing vitamin D levels and reducing inflammation, it is essential to balance sun exposure with the risk of skin damage, especially for individuals with autoimmune conditions that may make them more sensitive to sunlight.

Moderate Sun Exposure: Regular but moderate sun exposure (10-30 minutes a few times a week) can help maintain adequate vitamin D levels, especially for individuals at risk of autoimmune diseases. The amount of sun exposure needed varies depending on skin type, geographic location, and the time of year.

Vitamin D Supplementation: In regions with limited sunlight or for individuals who cannot tolerate sun exposure due to conditions like lupus, **vitamin D supplementation** can be an effective alternative for maintaining optimal vitamin D levels and reducing the risk of autoimmune flare-ups.

Avoiding Excessive Sun Exposure: Individuals with autoimmune conditions such as **SLE**, who may be photosensitive, should avoid prolonged sun exposure, especially during peak hours (10 a.m. to 4 p.m.). Using sunscreen and protective clothing can help mitigate the risks of sun-induced flare-ups while allowing controlled sun exposure to boost vitamin D levels.

The Future of Sunlight and Autoimmune Research

The relationship between sunlight, vitamin D, and autoimmune conditions continues to be a subject of research. Scientists are exploring how different levels of sunlight exposure and genetic factors influence the risk and progression of autoimmune diseases. Additionally, research is being conducted on the potential benefits of **phototherapy** (controlled exposure to UV light) for treating autoimmune-related inflammation, particularly in conditions like psoriasis.

Conclusion

Sunlight is pivotal in immune function, particularly in reducing inflammation associated with autoimmune diseases. By stimulating the production of vitamin D, sunlight helps regulate immune responses, balance T-cell activity, and inhibit the overproduction of pro-inflammatory cytokines. For individuals with autoimmune conditions like multiple sclerosis, rheumatoid arthritis, and lupus, maintaining adequate vitamin D levels through safe sun exposure or supplementation can significantly reduce inflammation and improve disease outcomes.

However, striking the right balance between sunlight exposure and skin protection is crucial, especially for those sensitive to UV light. As research advances, the connection between sunlight, vitamin D, and immune health offers promising insights into managing autoimmune disorders.

Seasonal Illnesses and Sunlight Deficiency: Why We Tend to Get Sicker in Winter When Sunlight Exposure is Lower

As the winter months arrive, many people experience an uptick in seasonal illnesses such as colds, flu, and other respiratory infections. One key factor contributing to this increase is the reduced exposure to sunlight during the colder months. Sunlight, mainly its role in stimulating **vitamin D production**, plays a crucial role in maintaining a healthy immune system. When sunlight exposure is limited during winter, it can weaken the body's defenses, making us more vulnerable to infections.

Reduced Sunlight and Lower Vitamin D Levels

Vitamin D, often called the "sunshine vitamin," is produced in the skin when exposed to **ultraviolet B (UVB)** rays from sunlight. This vitamin is essential for immune health, as it helps the body activate **T-cells** that are responsible for detecting and attacking pathogens like viruses and bacteria. Vitamin D also regulates immune responses, ensuring that inflammation is controlled and the body does not overreact to threats.

During the winter, the sun's rays are weaker, and people spend less time outdoors, reducing their exposure to UVB rays. This drop in sunlight exposure leads to lower vitamin D levels, which weakens the immune system's ability to fight off infections.

Weakened Immune Function: Low levels of vitamin D result in less effective activation of T-cells, meaning the immune system is slower to respond to invading pathogens. This leaves the body more susceptible to seasonal illnesses like the cold and flu.

Increased Inflammation: Vitamin D regulates inflammation in the body. A deficiency in vitamin D can result in an overactive immune response, leading to prolonged or excessive inflammation, which can exacerbate symptoms of illnesses.

The Role of Circadian Rhythm Disruption

Reduced sunlight in the winter also affects the body's **circadian rhythm**, the internal clock regulating sleep, wakefulness, and other essential bodily functions. Sunlight, remarkably morning light, helps regulate this rhythm by suppressing the production of **melatonin**, the hormone responsible for promoting sleep.

During the winter, shorter days and longer nights can disrupt the circadian rhythm, leading to **sleep disturbances** or reduced sleep quality. Poor sleep weakens the immune system, making it harder for the body to avoid infections.

Impact on the Immune System: Adequate sleep is critical for maintaining immune function. Sleep deprivation or poor-quality sleep suppresses the production of **cytokines** and proteins vital for immune responses. When the body doesn't get enough rest, it is less equipped to fight off illnesses.

Increased Stress and Cortisol Levels: Disruptions in the circadian rhythm can also lead to increased **cortisol** levels, the body's stress hormone. Elevated cortisol can weaken the immune system, further contributing to the likelihood of catching seasonal illnesses.

Increased Indoor Activity and Lack of Fresh Air

Another factor contributing to the rise in seasonal illnesses during winter is the shift in human behavior. People tend to spend more time indoors as temperatures drop, often in enclosed spaces with limited ventilation. This creates an environment where viruses and bacteria can spread more quickly.

Crowded Indoor Spaces: When more people gather indoors, the likelihood of exposure to airborne viruses like the flu or cold increases. Poor air circulation in heated spaces allows pathogens to linger in the air longer.

Lack of Fresh Air: Spending time outdoors in fresh air reduces the concentration of viruses in the environment. In contrast, heated indoor spaces can become breeding grounds for viruses, increasing the chance of transmission.

Seasonal Affective Disorder (SAD) and Immune Function

Seasonal Affective Disorder (SAD) is a type of depression that occurs during the winter months due to the lack of sunlight. People with SAD experience symptoms such as fatigue, sadness, and difficulty concentrating, but it can also have physical effects that impact the immune system.

Low Serotonin and Immune Health: Sunlight exposure increases the production of **serotonin**, a neurotransmitter that regulates mood. Low levels of serotonin, often experienced in SAD, can lead to feelings of fatigue and depression, which in turn can weaken the immune response and make it more difficult for the body to fight off infections.

Link to Vitamin D Deficiency: SAD is also associated with low vitamin D levels, as less sunlight is available to stimulate vitamin D production. This further weakens the immune system, making individuals with SAD more susceptible to seasonal illnesses.

Preventing Seasonal Illnesses Through Sunlight and Vitamin D

It is essential to compensate for the lack of sunlight exposure and its impact on the immune system to reduce the risk of seasonal illnesses during winter. Here are a few strategies to maintain immune function during the winter:

Vitamin D Supplementation: Vitamin **D supplements** can help maintain adequate vitamin D levels for those living in regions with limited winter sunlight. Experts recommend supplementing with **1,000 to 2,000 IU** of vitamin D daily, though the exact dosage may vary depending on individual needs and health conditions. Vitamin D-rich foods, such as fatty fish (salmon, mackerel), fortified milk, and eggs, can also help boost vitamin D levels.

Maximize Sun Exposure: Even though winter sunlight is weaker, spend time outdoors during the sunniest parts of the day. Aim to expose your skin to natural light for at least **10–30 minutes**, depending on your skin type and geographical location.

Maintain Healthy Sleep Patterns: Establishing a consistent sleep routine and getting enough sleep each night (7–9 hours for adults) helps maintain immune function and reduces the likelihood of illness. Try to expose yourself to natural light in the morning to regulate your circadian rhythm and improve sleep quality.

Exercise and Fresh Air: Regular physical activity, particularly outdoors, can help strengthen the immune system and improve overall health. Even in colder months, try to get fresh air by walking or exercising outdoors.

Conclusion

The increase in seasonal illnesses during winter is closely linked to reduced sunlight exposure, leading to lower vitamin D levels, circadian rhythm disruptions, and increased time spent indoors. These factors weaken the immune system, making individuals more susceptible to infections like colds and the flu. Incorporating strategies such as vitamin D supplementation, maximizing sunlight exposure, and maintaining healthy sleep habits can bolster immune function and reduce the risk of getting sick during the colder months. Maintaining a balance between protecting against winter illnesses and optimizing sunlight exposure is critical to staying healthy throughout the season.

7

Sunlight's Impact on Cardiovascular Health

Sunlight and Blood Pressure: How UV Rays Release Nitric Oxide, Leading to Vasodilation and Lower Blood Pressure

The health benefits of sunlight go beyond mood and vitamin D production—it also plays a significant role in cardiovascular health, particularly in regulating **blood pressure**. Recent research has uncovered that exposure to **ultraviolet (UV) rays** from sunlight triggers the release of **nitric oxide (NO)** in the skin, which leads to **vasodilation** (widening of blood vessels) and helps lower blood pressure. This process sheds light on how sunlight exposure can improve heart health and reduce the risk of hypertension.

The Role of Nitric Oxide in Blood Pressure Regulation

Nitric oxide (NO) is a molecule produced naturally in the body that acts as a potent **vasodilator**. It helps relax and widen blood vessels, allowing blood to flow more easily and reducing the pressure on artery walls. Nitric oxide is crucial for maintaining **vascular health**, and its release is associated with lower blood pressure and improved circulation.

Vasodilation: When nitric oxide is released, it signals the smooth muscles around the blood vessels to relax, causing the vessels to expand. This reduces the resistance to blood flow, lowering overall blood pressure.

Improved Blood Flow: Nitric oxide promotes vasodilation, ensuring that blood circulates more efficiently, delivering oxygen and nutrients to tissues and organs while reducing strain on the heart.

How UV Rays Trigger Nitric Oxide Release

While nitric oxide is produced in various body parts, including the blood vessels, research has shown that **UV exposure** from sunlight can also stimulate its release from **stores in the skin**. This process occurs independently of vitamin D production and directly impacts blood pressure.

UV Rays and the Skin: When exposed to **ultraviolet A (UVA) rays**, nitric oxide stored in the skin is released into the bloodstream. UVA rays penetrate the skin and trigger the breakdown of nitrosothiol compounds, which release nitric oxide. Once released into the blood, nitric oxide causes vasodilation, leading to a reduction in blood pressure.

Rapid Effects on Blood Pressure: Studies have shown that short-term exposure to UVA light can result in an immediate decrease in blood pressure, even without producing vitamin D. This suggests that sunlight's cardiovascular benefits are not solely tied to vitamin D synthesis but also to the direct effects of nitric oxide on the blood vessels.

Sunlight, Nitric Oxide, and Hypertension

Hypertension, or high blood pressure, is a leading risk factor for heart disease, stroke, and other cardiovascular conditions. Chronic hypertension occurs when blood pressure remains elevated over time, putting excessive strain on the heart and arteries. Sunlight exposure and the release of nitric oxide may help lower the risk of developing hypertension by promoting vasodilation and improving blood flow.

Natural Blood Pressure Regulation: Moderate sun exposure, particularly to UVA rays, can be a natural way to help regulate blood pressure. People living in regions with less sunlight, such as during winter months or in higher latitudes, are often at a higher risk of hypertension due to reduced nitric oxide release and vasodilation.

Potential Cardiovascular Benefits: Regular sunlight exposure may reduce the risk of cardiovascular diseases by helping to maintain healthy blood pressure levels. The release of nitric oxide, combined with other sunlight-related benefits like vitamin D production and improved mood, contributes to overall heart health.

The Balance Between Sun Exposure and Skin Health

While sunlight can have significant cardiovascular benefits by releasing nitric oxide, it is essential to balance sun exposure with the risk of skin damage, such as **sunburn** and **skin cancer**. Excessive exposure to UV rays, particularly UVB, can increase the risk of skin cancer, so it's crucial to enjoy sunlight safely.

Moderate Sun Exposure: To benefit from nitric oxide release without risking skin damage, it's recommended to get **10–30 minutes** of sunlight exposure several times a week, depending on your skin type and geographical location. This allows nitric oxide release and blood pressure regulation without overexposure to harmful UV rays.

Sunscreen Use: While sunscreen helps protect the skin from UVB rays that cause sunburn and increase cancer risk, it may also block some UVA rays responsible for nitric oxide release. Using sunscreen strategically—applying it after a brief period of sun exposure—can help you reap the cardiovascular benefits of sunlight while minimizing skin cancer risks.

The Seasonal Impact on Blood Pressure

The relationship between sunlight and nitric oxide also explains why blood pressure tends to be lower during summer and higher during winter. In colder months, reduced sunlight exposure leads to less nitric oxide release, which can contribute to elevated blood pressure.

Winter Hypertension: In many people, blood pressure rises during the winter due to less sunlight exposure and increased vasoconstriction (narrowing of blood vessels). Supplementing vitamin D and finding ways to improve safe sun exposure during the colder months may help mitigate this seasonal rise in blood pressure.

Geographic Variations: People living in regions with consistently high sunlight exposure tend to have lower average blood pressure than those living in areas with less sunlight. This suggests that geographic location and access to sunlight affect cardiovascular health.

Other Factors Influencing Blood Pressure

While sunlight and nitric oxide are essential factors in regulating blood pressure, they are part of a larger picture. Diet, physical activity, stress, and overall lifestyle habits are critical in maintaining healthy blood pressure levels. Incorporating safe sun exposure into a healthy lifestyle can support cardiovascular health, but it should be combined with other heart-healthy practices such as regular exercise and a balanced diet.

Conclusion

Sunlight profoundly affects blood pressure by triggering the release of **nitric oxide**, which promotes **vasodilation** and improves blood flow. This process helps lower blood pressure naturally, reducing the risk of hypertension and improving overall cardiovascular health. While sunlight can provide significant benefits for heart health, it's essential to enjoy it in moderation to avoid the risks of skin damage. Understanding the balance between safe sun exposure and its impact on nitric oxide and blood pressure can help people maintain healthy skin and heart.

Reduced Cardiovascular Risks: Understanding the link between regular sun exposure and lowered risk of heart attacks and strokes.

Reduced Cardiovascular Risks: Understanding the Link Between Regular Sun Exposure and Lowered Risk of Heart Attacks and Strokes

While excessive sun exposure can carry risks, **moderate, regular sun exposure** has been shown to provide significant health benefits, particularly in reducing the risk of **cardiovascular diseases** like **heart attacks** and **strokes**. Research indicates that sunlight exposure positively affects cardiovascular health by improving blood pressure regulation, enhancing vitamin D levels, and reducing inflammation. These factors work together to lower the overall risk of heart-related issues.

Sunlight and Nitric Oxide Release

One of the most important mechanisms through which sunlight impacts cardiovascular health is the release of **nitric oxide (NO)**. When skin is exposed to **ultraviolet A (UVA) rays**, it triggers the release of nitric oxide from stores in the skin into the bloodstream. Nitric oxide acts as a **vasodilator**, meaning it helps to relax and widen blood vessels, improving blood flow and reducing blood pressure.

Lower Blood Pressure: Nitric oxide release leads to **vasodilation**, reducing the resistance in blood vessels and allowing blood to flow more easily. This process lowers **blood pressure**, a significant risk factor for heart attacks and strokes. Studies have shown that people exposed to regular sunlight tend to have lower average blood pressure than those with limited sun exposure.

Improved Circulation: Nitric oxide widens the blood vessels, improving circulation and ensuring that oxygen and nutrients are efficiently delivered throughout the body. This reduction in vascular strain helps lower the risk of damage to the arteries, reducing the chance of heart disease.

Vitamin D and Heart Health

Sunlight stimulates vitamin D production, a crucial nutrient that plays a significant role in cardiovascular health. Vitamin D deficiency has been linked to an increased risk of **hypertension**, **atherosclerosis**, **heart attacks**, and **strokes**.

Inflammation Reduction: Vitamin D has anti-inflammatory properties, which can reduce the chronic inflammation that contributes to the development of cardiovascular diseases. High levels of inflammation can damage blood vessels and accelerate the progression of heart disease.

Improved Heart Function: Adequate vitamin D levels are associated with better heart function, as it helps regulate calcium in the blood, ensuring that the heart and muscles contract correctly. Deficiency in vitamin D can lead to calcification of blood vessels, a risk factor for atherosclerosis and heart attacks.

Sunlight and Cholesterol Management

Sunlight exposure may help manage **cholesterol levels**, mainly by converting **lousy cholesterol (LDL)** into **vitamin D**. Lower LDL cholesterol levels reduce the risk of plaque buildup in the arteries, a significant cause of heart attacks and strokes.

Cholesterol Conversion: When UVB rays from sunlight interact with the skin, they help convert cholesterol into vitamin D. This increases vitamin D levels and reduces LDL cholesterol, contributing to better cardiovascular health.

Reduced Plaque Formation: Lower cholesterol levels help prevent plaque formation in the arteries, reducing the risk of blockages that can lead to heart attacks and strokes.

Reduced Stress and Improved Heart Function

Sunlight exposure has been linked to lower levels of **cortisol**, the body's stress hormone. Elevated cortisol levels, particularly over long periods, can increase the risk of heart disease by raising blood pressure and contributing to inflammation. By reducing stress, sunlight promotes better cardiovascular health.

Lowered Cortisol Levels: Sunlight helps regulate the body's natural circadian rhythm, which can lower cortisol levels. Reduced stress is associated with improved heart function and a lower risk of hypertension, heart attacks, and strokes.

Enhanced Mood and Heart Health: Sunlight exposure boosts serotonin levels, improving mood and reducing feelings of depression or anxiety. Positive mental health contributes to reduced cardiovascular risk, as stress and mental health issues can negatively impact heart health.

Seasonal Variation in Heart Attack and Stroke Risks

Studies have shown that **heart attacks** and **strokes** are more common during the winter months when sunlight exposure is limited. This seasonal variation in cardiovascular risks is closely linked to reduced nitric oxide release, lower vitamin D levels, and increased stress during the darker months of the year.

Winter Hypertension: Blood pressure tends to be higher during the winter months due to reduced sunlight and lower nitric oxide production. This increase elevates the risk of cardiovascular events like heart attacks and strokes.

Vitamin D Deficiency in Winter: The lack of sunlight during the winter leads to lower vitamin D levels, increasing the risk of inflammation, higher cholesterol levels, and poorer heart function, all contributing to cardiovascular disease.

Guidelines for Safe Sun Exposure and Heart Health

While sunlight exposure offers significant cardiovascular benefits, it's important to strike a balance between gaining these advantages and protecting the skin from overexposure.

Excessive sun exposure can increase the risk of **skin cancer**, so moderation is key.

Moderate Sun Exposure: Aim for **10–30 minutes** of sunlight exposure several times a week, depending on skin type and geographic location. This amount of sun exposure can help promote nitric oxide release and boost vitamin D levels without risking skin damage.

Sun Protection: When spending extended time in the sun, wear sunscreen and protective clothing to shield your skin from harmful UVB rays. However, short periods of sun exposure without sunscreen can help you gain the cardiovascular benefits of sunlight safely.

Consider Vitamin D Supplements: For individuals who live in areas with limited sunlight or during winter months, **vitamin D supplements** may help maintain adequate levels of the vitamin, reducing the risk of cardiovascular diseases. Consult with a healthcare provider to determine the appropriate dosage.

Conclusion

Regular, moderate exposure to sunlight is crucial in reducing the risk of **heart attacks** and **strokes** by promoting the release of **nitric oxide**, improving blood pressure, and enhancing **vitamin D levels**. These factors contribute to better circulation, lower inflammation, and improved heart function, helping to prevent cardiovascular diseases. However, it's essential to balance sun exposure with protective measures to ensure long-term skin health. By incorporating safe sun habits into your daily routine, you can enjoy the heart-healthy benefits of sunlight while minimizing its risks.

Exploring Sunlight's Role in Metabolic Health: How Sunlight Can Reduce the Risk of Diabetes and Metabolic Syndrome

Emerging research suggests that moderate exposure to sunlight can improve **metabolic health**, potentially reducing the risk of **diabetes** and **metabolic syndrome**. These benefits are primarily linked to sunlight's effect on **vitamin D production, circadian rhythm regulation**, and **insulin sensitivity** and **inflammation** improvements. Understanding how sunlight contributes to metabolic health opens the door to natural ways of preventing and managing these chronic conditions.

The Role of Vitamin D in Metabolic Health

One primary way sunlight influences metabolic health is through the production of **vitamin D**, a hormone-like vitamin produced when the skin is exposed to **ultraviolet B (UVB)** rays from the sun. Vitamin D is critical in regulating **insulin** sensitivity, controlling **blood sugar levels**, and reducing inflammation, and it is vital for maintaining metabolic health.

Improving Insulin Sensitivity: Vitamin D enhances the body's ability to respond to insulin, the hormone that regulates blood sugar. It increases insulin receptors in cells, allowing more efficient glucose uptake from the bloodstream. This improved insulin sensitivity helps lower blood sugar levels and reduce the risk of developing **type 2 diabetes**.

Reducing Insulin Resistance: Vitamin D deficiency is associated with **insulin resistance**, a condition where the body's cells don't respond effectively to insulin, leading to elevated blood sugar levels. Insulin resistance is a critical component of metabolic syndrome and type 2 diabetes. Regular sunlight exposure, which boosts vitamin D levels, can help prevent or reduce insulin resistance.

Supporting Pancreatic Function: Vitamin D is also involved in maintaining the health of the **pancreatic beta cells**, which produce insulin. Adequate vitamin D levels help the pancreas function optimally, ensuring proper insulin secretion and blood sugar regulation.

Sunlight and Reduced Risk of Type 2 Diabetes

Studies have shown that individuals with **higher vitamin D levels**—often achieved through regular sun exposure—have a lower risk of developing type 2 diabetes. Here's how sunlight helps reduce this risk:

Glucose Regulation: Vitamin D plays a critical role in glucose metabolism by influencing the body's ability to regulate blood sugar. Individuals with adequate sunlight exposure tend to have lower fasting blood glucose levels, which helps prevent spikes in blood sugar and reduces the risk of type 2 diabetes.

Lower Risk of Obesity: Obesity is a significant risk factor for type 2 diabetes, and sunlight exposure has been linked to weight regulation. While the exact mechanisms are still being studied, sunlight exposure may influence **fat metabolism** and energy expenditure, helping to reduce body fat and lower the risk of diabetes.

Sunlight and Metabolic Syndrome

Metabolic syndrome is a cluster of conditions that increase the risk of heart disease, stroke, and type 2 diabetes. These conditions include high blood pressure, high blood sugar, excess body fat around the waist, and abnormal cholesterol levels. Sunlight exposure can help mitigate the risks associated with metabolic syndrome in several ways:

Improving Lipid Profiles: Studies have shown that sunlight exposure can improve **cholesterol** levels by converting lousy cholesterol

(**LDL**) into vitamin D, thereby reducing the risk of cardiovascular disease, closely linked to metabolic syndrome.

Regulating Blood Pressure: As mentioned earlier, sunlight exposure triggers the release of **nitric oxide**, which causes **vasodilation** and improves blood flow, leading to lower blood pressure. High blood pressure is one of the defining characteristics of metabolic syndrome, and sunlight's ability to help manage blood pressure naturally contributes to better metabolic health.

Weight Management and Fat Storage: Research suggests sunlight may influence **fat cells** and help regulate weight. Sunlight exposure has been linked to lower body fat and a more favorable **body mass index (BMI)**, which is essential in reducing metabolic syndrome risk.

Circadian Rhythm and Metabolic Health

Sunlight significantly regulates the body's **circadian rhythm**, the internal clock that governs sleep-wake cycles, hormone production, and metabolism. A well-functioning circadian rhythm is essential for maintaining metabolic health, as it influences when and how the body processes food and energy.

Impact on Insulin and Glucose Metabolism: The circadian rhythm affects insulin sensitivity, with the body being more insulin-sensitive in the morning and less so in the evening. Regular sunlight exposure, particularly in the morning, helps keep the circadian rhythm aligned, optimizing the body's ability to process glucose efficiently throughout the day. Disruptions in circadian rhythms—such as insufficient sunlight or irregular sleep patterns—can lead to **insulin resistance** and an increased risk of metabolic disorders.

Sleep and Metabolic Health: Poor sleep is linked to higher risks of obesity, insulin resistance, and metabolic syndrome. Sunlight exposure during the day, especially in the morning, promotes better sleep by regulating melatonin production, a hormone that governs sleep cycles.

Better sleep quality helps maintain metabolic balance and supports overall health.

Sunlight and Inflammation Reduction

Chronic **inflammation** is a hallmark of metabolic syndrome and diabetes. It contributes to insulin resistance, weight gain, and cardiovascular risk. Vitamin D, produced through sunlight exposure, is critical in reducing inflammation.

Anti-Inflammatory Effects: Vitamin D has been shown to reduce the production of **pro-inflammatory cytokines**, proteins that promote inflammation while increasing **anti-inflammatory cytokines**. This helps protect tissues from the damaging effects of chronic inflammation, improving overall metabolic function.

Immune Modulation: Sunlight's influence on the immune system, particularly its ability to enhance **T-cell function**, can help manage inflammation in the body. By reducing chronic inflammation, sunlight helps protect against the metabolic imbalances that lead to type 2 diabetes and metabolic syndrome.

Seasonal Variation in Metabolic Health

The risk of metabolic disorders tends to increase during winter when sunlight exposure is lower. This seasonal variation is mainly due to reduced vitamin D production and circadian rhythm disruptions, which contribute to weight gain, insulin resistance, and metabolic syndrome.

Winter Weight Gain: Many people experience weight gain during the winter months, partly due to lower physical activity levels but also because of reduced sunlight exposure. This weight gain can exacerbate insulin resistance and increase the risk of metabolic syndrome.

Vitamin D Supplementation: During the winter, when natural sunlight is limited, vitamin D supplements may help maintain metabolic health. Supplementing with vitamin D has been shown to improve insulin sensitivity and reduce inflammation, supporting metabolic function even during low sunlight exposure.

Practical Guidelines for Safe Sunlight Exposure and Metabolic Health

While sunlight provides significant benefits for metabolic health, it's essential to enjoy it safely to avoid the risks of overexposure, such as sunburn or skin cancer.

Aim for Moderate Sun Exposure: Try to spend **10–30 minutes** in sunlight several times a week, depending on your skin type, location, and the time of year. Exposing larger areas of the skin, such as the arms or legs, helps maximize vitamin D production.

Morning Sunlight for Circadian Health: Sunlight exposure helps regulate your circadian rhythm, improving sleep and metabolic function. Even 15 minutes of morning sunlight can have a positive impact.

Vitamin D Supplementation in Winter: For those living in areas with limited sunlight during winter, consider taking **vitamin D supplements** to maintain adequate levels and support metabolic health.

Conclusion

Sunlight is essential in maintaining **metabolic health** by improving **vitamin D** levels, enhancing **insulin sensitivity**, reducing **inflammation**, and regulating the **circadian rhythm**. These factors work together to reduce the risk of type 2 diabetes and metabolic syndrome.

Incorporating moderate sunlight exposure into daily life while balancing the need for skin protection can provide powerful metabolic benefits and help prevent chronic metabolic conditions. By understanding the connection between sunlight and metabolic health, we can use natural methods to improve overall well-being and reduce the risk of diabetes and related disorders.

8

The Importance of Sunlight for Children and Adolescents

Supporting Healthy Development: The Role of Sunlight in Bone Growth, Mental Health, and Immune Development in Children

Sunlight plays a vital role in children's healthy growth and development, impacting areas such as **bone health**, **mental well-being**, and **immune system function**. By stimulating the production of **vitamin D** and influencing biological rhythms, sunlight contributes significantly to children's physical and psychological health during crucial stages of development.

Sunlight and Bone Growth

One of the most well-known roles of sunlight in children's health is its contribution to **bone growth** through the production of **vitamin D**. When a child's skin is exposed to **ultraviolet B (UVB)** rays from sunlight, the body produces vitamin D, which is crucial for the absorption of **calcium** and **phosphorus**, minerals essential for building strong bones.

Vitamin D and Calcium Absorption:

Vitamin D facilitates calcium absorption from the diet into the bloodstream. Without adequate vitamin D, the body cannot effectively absorb calcium, leading to weak bones and the risk of developing rickets, a condition where bones become soft and deformed.

Preventing Bone Diseases: Children who do not get enough sunlight are at risk of **vitamin D deficiency**, which can impair bone mineralization and lead to conditions like **osteomalacia** and **osteoporosis** later in life. Regular exposure to sunlight during childhood helps ensure strong bones and reduces the risk of bone-related diseases as children grow.

Support During Growth Spurts: During periods of rapid growth, such as infancy and adolescence, children need higher calcium and vitamin D levels to support bone development. Ensuring they get sufficient sunlight is critical during these times.

Sunlight and Mental Health in Children

Sunlight significantly impacts children's **mental health** and well-being by regulating the production of neurotransmitters like **serotonin** and maintaining a healthy **circadian rhythm**. These factors contribute to emotional balance, mood stability, and mental health.

Boosting Serotonin Levels: Exposure to sunlight increases the production of **serotonin**, a neurotransmitter associated with happiness and well-being. Higher serotonin levels can help reduce feelings of anxiety, depression, and irritability, promoting a more positive mood in children. This is especially important in maintaining emotional balance and managing stress during development.

Preventing Mood Disorders: Lack of sunlight, particularly during the winter months, has been linked to **Seasonal Affective Disorder (SAD)** and other mood-related issues in children.

Regular exposure to sunlight can prevent these disorders and promote a more positive outlook and mental health.

Regulating the Circadian Rhythm: Sunlight exposure in the morning helps regulate the body's **circadian rhythm**, which governs sleep-wake cycles. A well-regulated circadian rhythm ensures better sleep quality, which is critical for children'schildren's development. Children who experience disruptions in their sleep due to poor circadian rhythm alignment may suffer from mood swings, cognitive difficulties, and behavioral issues.

Promoting Play and Physical Activity: Sunlight encourages children to spend more time outdoors, promoting physical activity, which is essential for mental and physical development. Outdoor play stimulates creativity and social interaction, enhances cognitive functioning, and reduces stress.

Sunlight and Immune Development

Sunlight plays a crucial role in developing a child's **immune system**, helping to strengthen the body's defenses against infections and illnesses. This is primarily due to sunlight's role in producing **vitamin D**, which supports immune function.

Vitamin D and Immune Support: Vitamin D is crucial for the proper functioning of the immune system. It helps activate **T-cells**, which are essential for detecting and fighting infections.

Adequate vitamin D levels support a robust immune response, reducing the risk of diseases like colds, flu, and other respiratory illnesses in children.

Reducing the Risk of Autoimmune Conditions: Vitamin D

regulates the immune system and reduces chronic inflammation, which may help lower the risk of developing **autoimmune conditions** such as **type 1 diabetes** or **juvenile arthritis**. Ensuring that children get enough sunlight may help protect them from such conditions later in life.

Preventing Respiratory Infections: Studies have shown that children with low vitamin D levels are more prone to **respiratory infections** and illnesses, especially during the winter when sunlight is reduced. Regular sun exposure helps maintain adequate vitamin D levels, reducing the incidence and severity of such infections.

Safe Sun Exposure for Children

While sunlight offers numerous health benefits, it's essential to balance sun exposure with the need for skin protection, especially in children. Overexposure to sunlight, particularly UVB rays, can increase the risk of **sunburn** and long-term skin damage, such as **skin cancer**.

Moderate Sun Exposure: Children should aim to get **10–30 minutes** of sun exposure several times a week, depending on their skin type, location, and time of year. This amount of sunlight is generally sufficient to boost vitamin D production without increasing the risk of sunburn.

Sun Protection: During extended periods outdoors, especially during peak sunlight hours (10 a.m. to 4 p.m.), it's essential to use **sunscreen**, hats, and protective clothing to shield children's skin from harmful UV rays. Sunscreen should be applied after a brief period of direct exposure to allow for some vitamin D production before complete protection is used.

Maximize Morning Sunlight: Morning sunlight helps regulate the circadian rhythm and promotes serotonin production, supporting sleep and mood. Encourage outdoor activities early in the day for optimal health benefits.

Seasonal Impact on Development

During the winter months, many children experience reduced exposure to sunlight due to shorter days and colder weather, which can impact their **vitamin D levels, immune function,** and **mental health.**

Vitamin D Supplementation: In regions with limited winter sunlight or for children who spend most of their time indoors, **vitamin D supplements** can help maintain adequate levels of the vitamin. It's recommended to consult with a healthcare provider to determine appropriate supplementation based on the child's age and health needs.

Encouraging Outdoor Activity: Even in colder months, it's essential to encourage children to spend time outdoors to reap the benefits of natural light and physical activity. Bundle them appropriately and aim for midday outdoor play when the sun is brightest.

Conclusion

Sunlight promotes healthy development in children, from supporting strong **bone growth** and **mental health** to enhancing **immune system function**. Ensuring that children get regular, moderate exposure to sunlight is essential for their physical and psychological well-being, especially during periods of rapid growth and development. By balancing safe sun exposure with protection, parents can help foster healthy habits and support the overall development of their children.

Vitamin D Deficiency in Childhood: The Rise of Rickets and Other Health Issues Due to Lack of Sunlight

Vitamin D deficiency in childhood is a growing concern, as it can lead to serious health issues, most notably **rickets**—a condition characterized by weakened, soft bones that can lead to deformities and stunted growth. The root cause of this deficiency is often a lack of adequate **sunlight exposure**, which is critical for vitamin D synthesis. As more children spend time indoors and face environmental or cultural factors limiting sun exposure, vitamin D deficiency is becoming increasingly prevalent, raising the risk of various developmental and health problems.

The Importance of Vitamin D in Childhood

Vitamin D plays a crucial role in children's growth and development, particularly in maintaining healthy **bones** and a strong **immune system**. Without sufficient vitamin D, children cannot properly absorb **calcium** and **phosphorus**, essential minerals for bone formation and overall health.

Bone Growth and Strength: Vitamin D helps regulate calcium levels in the body by promoting its absorption from food. This process ensures that bones grow strong and healthy. Children risk developing weak bones without adequate vitamin D, leading to conditions like rickets.

Immune System Support: Vitamin D also supports the immune system, helping children avoid infections. Deficiency can make children more susceptible to illnesses such as colds, respiratory diseases, and, in some cases, autoimmune disorders.

The Rise of Rickets

Rickets is a disease that results from a severe deficiency of vitamin D, calcium, or phosphate, leading to softening and weakening of bones. It primarily affects children during their growth spurts, when they need these nutrients most for bone development. Once a common disease in the early 20th century, rickets disappeared mainly due to improved access to fortified foods and sunlight exposure. Still, it is now making a comeback due to modern lifestyle changes.

Symptoms of Rickets: Rickets include bone pain or tenderness, delayed growth, muscle weakness, and skeletal deformities such as bowed legs or thickened wrists and ankles. In severe cases, children may develop **dental issues** due to poor enamel formation and **skeletal abnormalities** that can become permanent if left untreated.

Causes of Rickets: The primary cause of rickets is a lack of sunlight, which impairs the body's ability to produce vitamin D. In some cases, poor dietary intake of vitamin D or underlying medical conditions that affect vitamin D metabolism can also lead to rickets. However, the lack of regular sunlight exposure remains the most common cause.

Modern Factors Contributing to Vitamin D Deficiency in Children

The re-emergence of vitamin D deficiency and related health issues such as rickets can largely be attributed to modern lifestyle changes and environmental factors limiting children's sunlight exposure. These include:

Increased Indoor Activities: Today, many children spend most of their time indoors, often in front of screens. Whether for entertainment or school, the amount of time children spend outside, where they could naturally produce vitamin D from sunlight, has significantly decreased.

Sunscreen Use: While sunscreen protects against skin cancer and sunburn, excessive use can block the UVB rays necessary for vitamin D synthesis. Children who wear sunscreen all the time or who avoid direct sunlight may not produce enough vitamin D.

Urban Living and Pollution: In densely populated urban areas, tall buildings and air pollution can block sunlight, reducing children's access to natural UVB rays. Air pollution also reduces the amount of UVB radiation that reaches the earth's surface, further limiting vitamin D production in children living in these environments.

Geographic Location: Children living in higher latitudes or regions with long winters and limited sunlight, such as northern Europe or Canada, are at greater risk of vitamin D deficiency due to fewer opportunities for sun exposure throughout the year.

Cultural and Religious Practices: In some cultures, children wear clothing that covers most of the skin, limiting exposure to sunlight. While this clothing may be necessary for cultural or religious reasons, it can contribute to vitamin D deficiency if not balanced with dietary sources of vitamin D or supplementation.

Other Health Issues Linked to Vitamin D Deficiency

Beyond rickets, vitamin D deficiency in childhood is linked to several other health issues, both immediate and long-term:

Delayed Growth and Development: Vitamin D deficiency can lead to delayed physical growth, especially in height, and can impact a child's ability to reach developmental milestones.

Weakened Immune System: A lack of vitamin D weakens the immune system, making children more prone to infections such as colds and the flu and respiratory issues like bronchitis and pneumonia.

Increased Risk of Chronic Diseases: Research suggests that children with low levels of vitamin D may have an increased risk of developing chronic diseases later in life, such as **type 1 diabetes, asthma, cardiovascular diseases**, and even **autoimmune disorders**.

Poor Dental Health: Vitamin D deficiency can lead to dental problems, including delayed tooth eruption and enamel defects, which may increase the risk of cavities and gum diseases.

Preventing Vitamin D Deficiency in Children

Preventing vitamin D deficiency in children requires a balance of safe sun exposure, proper nutrition, and, in some cases, supplementation:

Safe Sun Exposure: Encouraging children to spend time outdoors in the sunlight is one of the most effective ways to ensure they get enough vitamin D. Aim for **10–30 minutes** of sun exposure a few times a week, depending on skin type and geographic location. This exposure is most effective in the middle of the day when the sun is strongest.

Dietary Sources of Vitamin D: Along with sunlight, ensure children are consuming foods rich in vitamin D, such as:

Fatty fish (salmon, tuna, mackerel) Egg yolks Fortified dairy products and plant-based milks Fortified cereals Cod liver oil

Vitamin D Supplementation: Supplementation may be necessary in cases where children cannot get enough sunlight or dietary vitamin D. Pediatricians often recommend **400–600 IU** of vitamin D daily, depending on the child's age, overall health, and risk factors.

Education on Sunscreen Use: While sunscreen is crucial for preventing skin damage, it is also important to balance its use to allow for some natural vitamin D production. Parents should be educated on allowing short sun exposure before applying sunscreen, particularly in the early morning or late afternoon when UV rays are less intense.

The Role of Public Health and Awareness

Raising awareness about vitamin D deficiency and its consequences is essential in preventing a resurgence of conditions like rickets. Public health campaigns that promote safe sun exposure educate families about the importance of vitamin D, and encourage regular health check-ups for children can help combat this preventable deficiency.

Conclusion

Vitamin D deficiency in children, often due to a lack of adequate sunlight exposure, is leading to a resurgence of health issues like **rickets** and other developmental problems. The importance of vitamin D in **bone health**, **immune function**, and overall growth cannot be overstated.

Addressing this deficiency through safe sun exposure, dietary adjustments, and supplementation where necessary can prevent long-term health consequences and ensure children grow strong and healthy. By understanding the causes and solutions, parents, educators, and healthcare professionals can work together to reduce the risk of vitamin D deficiency and its associated health issues.

Encouraging Outdoor Play for Healthy Growth: How Outdoor Activities in Natural Light Contribute to Overall Well-Being

Outdoor play is essential to a child's healthy growth and development. Engaging in outdoor activities, especially in natural light, offers numerous physical, mental, and social benefits that contribute to overall well-being. From improving physical fitness to enhancing emotional resilience, spending time outdoors promotes a balanced and healthy lifestyle that is crucial for children. Here are the key ways in which outdoor play in natural light supports children's development:

Physical Health and Bone Development

One of the most immediate benefits of outdoor play is improved **physical fitness**. Outdoor environments naturally encourage children to be more active, helping to improve their **strength**, **coordination**, and **balance**. Additionally, exposure to sunlight plays a crucial role in supporting **bone health** by promoting vitamin D production.

Increased Physical Activity: Running, jumping, climbing, and engaging in outdoor play help children develop muscle strength, improve cardiovascular health, and maintain a healthy body weight. Regular physical activity reduces the risk of childhood obesity and related health issues such as type 2 diabetes and high blood pressure.

Vitamin D and Bone Growth: Sunlight exposure triggers the production of vitamin D in the skin, essential for **calcium absorption** and healthy **bone development**. Adequate vitamin D levels help prevent **rickets** and other bone-related disorders in children. Encouraging outdoor play in natural light ensures children get the necessary vitamin D to support their growing bones.

Boosting Mental Health and Emotional Well-Being

Spending time outdoors in natural light can positively affect children's **mental health** and **emotional well-being**. Sunlight stimulates the production of **serotonin**, a hormone that enhances mood and promotes happiness and calmness. Outdoor play can help children manage stress, anxiety, and even depression.

Improved Mood and Reduced Anxiety: Exposure to sunlight helps boost serotonin levels, leading to improved mood and reduced symptoms of anxiety and depression. Outdoor play allows children to enjoy time in nature, which has been shown to reduce stress and promote a sense of calm.

Enhanced Creativity and Imagination: The natural environment offers limitless opportunities for imaginative play. Whether building a fort, pretending to be an explorer, or playing games, children are more likely to engage in creative play outdoors, fostering cognitive development and problem-solving skills.

Connection to Nature and Mindfulness: Outdoors allows children to connect with nature, encouraging mindfulness and appreciation for their surroundings. This connection can foster a sense of peace and balance, contributing to emotional resilience and mental clarity.

Supporting Cognitive Development and Learning

Outdoor play encourages **curiosity** and exploration, which supports **cognitive development**. Engaging with the natural world can enhance children's understanding of the environment, promote critical thinking, and encourage a love for learning.

Improved Focus and Attention: Outdoor play helps improve children's ability to concentrate and focus. Studies have shown that children who spend time in nature have better attention spans and are more engaged in learning tasks when they return indoors. This is especially beneficial for children with **attention deficit hyperactivity disorder (ADHD)**, as outdoor activities can help them regulate their energy levels and improve focus.

Hands-On Learning: Outdoor environments provide opportunities for hands-on learning, whether observing wildlife, building with natural materials, or exploring different textures and terrains. These experiences foster a deeper understanding of science, geography, and social studies, offering practical learning opportunities that complement classroom education.

Social Skills and Emotional Intelligence

Outdoor play often involves **group activities**, which provide children with opportunities to develop essential **social skills** such as **teamwork**, **communication**, and **empathy**. Playing with peers in a natural environment encourages cooperation, negotiation, and problem-solving in a social context.

Improving Communication: Outdoor play encourages children to communicate more effectively with their peers, whether organizing a game, resolving conflicts, or working together on a project. These interactions help build communication skills and foster strong friendships.

Building Emotional Intelligence: Outdoor play helps children develop **emotional intelligence** by encouraging them to express their feelings, empathize with others, and navigate social challenges. Children who engage in outdoor group play are better equipped to manage their emotions and build healthy relationships.

Encouraging Risk-Taking and Resilience: Outdoor play often involves elements of controlled risk, such as climbing trees, jumping over obstacles, or balancing on logs. These activities help children develop resilience and confidence, teaching them to assess risks and cope with challenges in a safe environment.

Circadian Rhythm and Sleep Quality

Natural light is essential for regulating the body's **circadian rhythm**, the internal clock that governs sleep-wake cycles. Outdoor play, particularly in the morning, helps children maintain healthy sleep patterns by aligning their circadian rhythm with natural daylight.

Better Sleep: Exposure to sunlight during the day helps regulate melatonin production, a hormone that promotes sleep. Children who spend more time outdoors are more likely to fall asleep quickly and enjoy a deeper, more restful sleep.

Improved Behavior and Focus: A well-regulated circadian rhythm enhances sleep quality, daytime behavior, and cognitive function. Children who get enough natural light and rest are more focused, less irritable, and better able to handle the demands of school and social interactions.

Fostering a Lifelong Love of Physical Activity

Encouraging outdoor play from an early age helps instill a **love for physical activity** and healthy living, which can continue into adolescence and adulthood. Children who regularly engage in outdoor play are more likely to develop habits of being active, which supports long-term health and well-being.

Building Healthy Habits: Outdoor play encourages children to engage in physical activities like running, cycling, hiking, and sports, which can foster a lifelong appreciation for exercise. Active children are more likely to grow into active adults who prioritize physical fitness as part of a healthy lifestyle.

Reducing Screen Time: Encouraging outdoor play helps minimize screen time, which can negatively affect physical and mental health. Time spent in front of screens has been linked to sedentary behavior, poor sleep, and decreased social interaction. Outdoor play offers a natural, engaging alternative to screen-based activities.

Encouraging Independence and Problem-Solving

Outdoor play often involves challenges that require **independent thinking** and **problem-solving**. Whether figuring out how to build a structure or navigating a natural obstacle, children develop independence and self-confidence through outdoor exploration.

Developing Problem-Solving Skills: Outdoor play often presents children with challenges that encourage creative thinking and resourcefulness. Children learn to make decisions, adapt to new situations, and find solutions to obstacles, all contributing to cognitive and emotional growth.

Building Confidence and Autonomy: As children explore the outdoors and tackle challenges independently, they build confidence in their abilities and develop a sense of autonomy. This fosters a strong sense of self-esteem and personal accomplishment.

Conclusion

Outdoor play in natural light is essential for children's **healthy growth** and **well-being**. It supports physical development through **bone growth** and fitness, improves **mental health** by enhancing mood and reducing anxiety, and fosters **social skills** and **emotional intelligence** through group play and interactions. By encouraging children to spend time outdoors, we can help them develop essential life skills, support their cognitive and emotional growth, and instill healthy habits that will benefit them for years.

2

Sunlight and Aging Gracefully

The Role of Sunlight in Healthy Aging: How Adequate Sunlight Supports Strong Bones, a Healthy Immune System, and Mental Sharpness

Maintaining optimal health becomes increasingly important as we age, and sunlight plays a crucial role in supporting various aspects of healthy aging. Adequate exposure to sunlight has numerous benefits for seniors, promoting strong bones, a robust immune system, and mental sharpness. Below, we explore how sunlight contributes to healthy aging through these critical areas.

Supporting Strong Bones: The Role of Vitamin D in Bone Health

As people age, bone density naturally decreases, increasing the risk of osteoporosis, fractures, and other bone-related conditions. Adequate sunlight exposure helps counter this by promoting vitamin D synthesis, a nutrient essential for maintaining strong bones.

Vitamin D and Calcium Absorption: Sunlight stimulates the skin to produce vitamin D, which aids the body's calcium absorption from the diet. Calcium is vital for maintaining bone density and strength. Without enough vitamin D, the body cannot absorb calcium efficiently, leading to brittle bones and a higher risk of fractures.

Preventing Osteoporosis: Osteoporosis, a condition characterized by weak and porous bones, is more common in older adults, particularly women after menopause. Sunlight exposure helps mitigate the risk of osteoporosis by ensuring adequate vitamin D levels, which support bone regeneration and strength.

Falls and Fracture Prevention: Research has shown that individuals with adequate vitamin D levels tend to have stronger bones and muscles, which can help prevent falls and fractures—common issues among the elderly. To reduce these risks, a combination of vitamin D, calcium, and safe sunlight exposure is recommended.

Strengthening the Immune System: Sunlight's Role in Immune Health

Older adults become more vulnerable to infections and diseases as their immune systems weaken. Sunlight exposure can help strengthen the immune system through its role in vitamin D production.

Boosting Immune Response: Vitamin D enhances the function of **T-cells** and **macrophages**, key immune system components. These cells defend the body against pathogens, including viruses and bacteria. Higher vitamin D levels have been linked to a reduced risk of infections such as the flu, pneumonia, and respiratory illnesses, which can be particularly severe for older adults.

Reducing Inflammation and Autoimmune Risks: Sunlight exposure may also help modulate the immune system's inflammatory response. Chronic inflammation is a risk factor for many age-related diseases, including cardiovascular diseases and autoimmune disorders like rheumatoid arthritis. Vitamin D's anti-inflammatory properties can help regulate the immune system and reduce excessive inflammation, contributing to healthier aging.

Enhancing Mental Sharpness: Sunlight and Cognitive Health: Cognitive decline, including memory loss and decreased mental sharpness, is a common concern for aging adults. Adequate sunlight exposure can play a vital role in maintaining brain health and mental acuity as we age

Sunlight, Serotonin, and Mood: Sunlight helps regulate the production of **serotonin**, a neurotransmitter that impacts mood, energy levels, and cognitive function. Higher serotonin levels are associated with improved mood, focus, and clarity. In contrast, low serotonin levels can lead to depression and cognitive difficulties. Regular sunlight exposure can help stabilize mood and enhance mental sharpness

Preventing Seasonal Affective Disorder (SAD): Older adults, especially those in regions with long winters, may experience **Seasonal Affective Disorder (SAD)** due to reduced sunlight exposure. SAD is linked to decreased serotonin and can cause symptoms of depression and cognitive sluggishness. Light therapy or regular exposure to natural sunlight during the day can help mitigate these effects and improve mental clarity.

Sunlight and Sleep-Wake Cycles (Circadian Rhythms): Adequate sunlight exposure is critical for maintaining the body's **circadian rhythms**, the internal clock that regulates sleep-wake cycles. As people age, disruptions in circadian rhythms can lead to insomnia, fatigue, and cognitive impairment. Sunlight exposure, particularly in the morning, helps synchronize these rhythms, promoting better sleep and mental alertness throughout the day.

Reduced Risk of Dementia and Cognitive Decline: Some

research suggests that maintaining adequate vitamin D levels through sunlight exposure may reduce the risk of cognitive decline and dementia in older adults. Vitamin D receptors are present in areas of the brain involved in memory and cognitive processing, and studies have shown that vitamin D deficiency may be linked to an increased risk of Alzheimer's disease and other forms of dementia.

Conclusion: Sunlight as a Key Element in Healthy Aging

Regular, moderate sunlight exposure in daily life is essential to healthy aging. Sunlight plays a multifaceted role in supporting older adults' overall health and well-being by promoting solid bones, bolstering the immune system, and enhancing mental sharpness. While balancing sun exposure with skin protection is crucial, ensuring that seniors get enough natural light can make a significant difference in maintaining vitality and quality of life as they age.

Preventing Osteoporosis and Cognitive Decline: The Importance of Sunlight for Elderly Individuals

As people age, their risk of developing osteoporosis and experiencing cognitive decline increases. Adequate sunlight exposure is vital in mitigating these risks, primarily due to its role in promoting vitamin D synthesis, which is essential for bone health and cognitive function.

Below, we explore how sunlight helps protect against osteoporosis and supports mental health in elderly individuals.

Preventing Osteoporosis: Sunlight's Role in Bone Health

Osteoporosis is when bones become weak and brittle, making them more susceptible to fractures. It is widespread in older adults, especially postmenopausal women. One of the main contributors to osteoporosis is **vitamin D deficiency**, often due to inadequate sunlight exposure.

Vitamin D and Calcium Absorption: Vitamin D is essential for the body to absorb calcium from the diet. Calcium is a critical mineral for bone strength; without enough vitamin D, the body cannot efficiently absorb or utilize it. As a result, bones can become thin, weak, and prone to fractures. Sunlight exposure stimulates the skin to produce vitamin D, which supports proper calcium absorption and bone mineralization, helping to prevent osteoporosis.

Maintaining Bone Density: As individuals age, their bones naturally lose density.

Sunlight-derived vitamin D helps slow down this loss by supporting bone regeneration. Regular sun exposure can help elderly individuals maintain bone mass and reduce the likelihood of fractures. This is particularly important for older adults, as broken bones can lead to prolonged immobility and reduced quality of life.

Fracture Prevention: Older people are at a higher risk for falls, which can result in fractures, especially in individuals with osteoporosis. Adequate vitamin D levels contribute to stronger bones and muscles, improving balance and reducing the risk of falls and fractures. Studies show that vitamin D supplementation, combined with sunlight exposure, can help decrease the incidence of fractures in older adults.

Promoting Cognitive Function: Sunlight and Brain Health

As the population ages, **cognitive decline** and diseases like dementia and Alzheimer's become increasingly prevalent. Sunlight exposure, through its role in vitamin D production and circadian rhythm regulation, can help protect cognitive function and delay the onset of age-related cognitive impairments.

Vitamin D and Cognitive Health: The brain has vitamin D receptors, particularly in areas associated with memory and learning. Adequate vitamin D levels support **neuroplasticity**, the brain's ability to form new connections and maintain healthy brain function. Research has shown that vitamin D deficiency is associated with an increased risk of **dementia** and **cognitive decline**. By maintaining sufficient vitamin D levels through sunlight exposure, elderly individuals may reduce their risk of cognitive impairment.

Preventing Alzheimer's Disease: Some studies suggest that vitamin D may play a protective role against **Alzheimer's disease** by helping to reduce inflammation in the brain and clearing amyloid plaques, which are believed to contribute to the development of Alzheimer's. Ensuring that elderly individuals get enough sunlight to maintain optimal vitamin D levels could be a crucial factor in lowering the risk of developing Alzheimer's and other forms of dementia.

Regulating Circadian Rhythms and Sleep: Sunlight exposure helps regulate the body's **circadian rhythms**, which control the sleep-wake cycle. Disruptions in circadian rhythms are linked to poor sleep, cognitive decline, and an increased risk of dementia in elderly individuals. Sunlight, particularly in the morning, helps synchronize these rhythms, promoting better sleep quality and supporting cognitive health. Elderly individuals who receive regular sunlight exposure often experience improved mental alertness and cognitive function.

Mood and Mental Clarity: Sunlight boosts the production of **serotonin**, a neurotransmitter that affects mood, focus, and mental clarity. Low serotonin levels are associated with depression and cognitive sluggishness, particularly in older adults. By maintaining serotonin levels through regular sun exposure, elderly individuals can experience enhanced mood and cognitive sharpness, reducing the likelihood of depression, which is often a contributing factor to cognitive decline.

Conclusion: Sunlight's Dual Role in Protecting Bone and Brain Health

For elderly individuals, sunlight exposure is a simple yet powerful tool for maintaining physical and cognitive health. By promoting vitamin D production, sunlight helps protect against osteoporosis by supporting bone density and calcium absorption. Additionally, sunlight is critical in promoting cognitive function by regulating circadian rhythms, enhancing mood, and potentially reducing the risk of dementia and Alzheimer's.

Balancing adequate sunlight exposure with skin protection is essential, but incorporating regular time outdoors in the sunlight can provide long-term health benefits, allowing elderly individuals to maintain strong bones and a sharp mind as they age.

Moderate Sun Exposure for Longevity: Studies Linking Regular, Moderate Sun Exposure to Increased Lifespan and Quality of Life

Sunlight has been recognized for its numerous health benefits, and research increasingly suggests that regular, moderate sun exposure can contribute to both increased lifespan and enhanced quality of life. Exposure to sunlight provides a range of physiological advantages, such as promoting vitamin D production, regulating circadian rhythms, and improving mood—all of which can positively impact longevity and overall well-being.

Increased Lifespan: The Link Between Sunlight and Longevity

Several studies have shown a correlation between moderate sun exposure and increased lifespan. Individuals who regularly spend time in the sun appear to live longer, partly due to sunlight's various health benefits.

One significant study found that people with regular sun exposure had a lower risk of death from all causes, particularly from cardiovascular diseases. Sunlight promotes cardiovascular health, which may be a critical factor in extending lifespan. Additionally, moderate sun exposure is believed to reduce the risk of certain chronic diseases, such as diabetes, autoimmune disorders, and some cancers, which are significant contributors to early mortality.

Furthermore, sunlight supports the immune system, helping the body fight infections and illnesses that can shorten lifespan, especially in older adults. Sunlight's ability to reduce inflammation and enhance immune function may help explain the link between moderate sun exposure and increased longevity.

Enhanced Quality of Life: The Role of Sunlight in Physical and Mental Well-Being

Regular sunlight exposure can greatly enhance quality of life by supporting physical health and mental well-being, in addition to increasing lifespan.

Sunlight is known to boost the production of serotonin, a neurotransmitter associated with happiness and well-being. Higher serotonin levels improve mood and mental clarity, helping to reduce symptoms of depression and anxiety. Regular exposure to natural light can also help prevent mood disorders like Seasonal Affective Disorder (SAD), which can significantly affect quality of life, particularly in regions with long winters and limited sunlight.

Moreover, sunlight is critical in regulating circadian rhythms, which control sleep patterns. Properly regulated circadian rhythms result in better sleep, essential for cognitive function, physical health, and vitality. Improved sleep leads to better memory, reduced stress, and enhanced overall health

Physical health also benefits from sunlight exposure. Sunlight helps the body produce vitamin D, crucial for maintaining strong bones. This is particularly important for preventing osteoporosis and fractures in older adults, which can severely impact mobility and independence. By promoting more robust bones and muscles, moderate sun exposure helps individuals stay active and engaged, improving their quality of life as they age.

The Balance of Moderate Sun Exposure and Skin Protection

While moderate sun exposure offers many health benefits, it's crucial to balance it with proper skin protection to avoid risks such as sunburn, premature aging, and skin cancer. Experts recommend short periods of sun exposure, typically 10 to 30 minutes a few times a week, depending on skin type, to gain the benefits without overexposure. Sunscreen, protective clothing, and seeking shade during peak sunlight can reduce risks while allowing individuals to benefit from sunlight.

Individuals may need more sun exposure in areas with limited sunlight, particularly during winter. In such cases, vitamin D supplementation can help maintain the positive health effects of sunlight exposure.

Conclusion: Sunlight's Role in Longevity and Quality of Life

Moderate, regular sun exposure promotes longevity and a higher quality of life. By improving physical health, enhancing mood, and supporting immune function, sunlight contributes to long-term vitality and well-being. While sun protection remains important, incorporating sensible amounts of sunlight into daily life can help individuals live longer, healthier, and more fulfilling lives.

10

Practical Ways to Safely Incorporate Sunlight into Your Life

O ptimal Times for Sun Exposure: The best times of day are when you can get the benefits of sunlight without the risks of overexposure.

The optimal times for sun exposure, when you can get the benefits of sunlight without the risks of overexposure, generally fall during the early morning and late afternoon hours. Here's why:

Morning Sunlight (Before 10 AM)

The UV index is typically lower, reducing the risk of sunburn.

Exposure to morning sunlight helps with the production of **vitamin D**, which is essential for bone health and immune function.

The early sunlight also helps regulate your **circadian rhythm**, improving sleep patterns by encouraging melatonin production later in the day.

Late Afternoon Sunlight (After 4 PM)

Similar to morning hours, the UV index is lower in the late afternoon, reducing the risk of skin damage.

You still get the benefits of natural light without the harsh intensity of midday UV rays.

This time can also help to boost **mood** and reduce stress through increased serotonin levels.

Key Considerations:

It's crucial to avoid midday exposure (10 AM - 4 PM) when the sun's rays are strongest. This is a responsible choice that significantly reduces the risk of skin damage, aging, and skin cancer.Always wear sunscreen if you plan on extended time in the sun, even during these optimal hours, especially if you have fair skin or are sensitive to sun exposure.

By being mindful of these times, you can confidently enjoy the health benefits of sunlight while minimizing harmful effects. This reassurance is a key part of maintaining your health and wellness.

Sunlight, Sunscreen, and Skin Protection: How to balance sun exposure with sunscreen to prevent damage.

Balancing sun exposure with sunscreen to prevent skin damage involves understanding how to maximize the benefits of sunlight while minimizing risks like sunburn, premature aging, and skin cancer. Here are strategies to achieve this balance:

Understand Your Skin Type

Fair skin burns more efficiently and needs higher SPF sunscreen for more prolonged exposure, while **darker skin** provides more natural protection but is still vulnerable to UV damage.

All skin types need protection, but knowing your skin type helps you tailor your sun exposure and sunscreen use.

Optimal Sun Exposure

Moderation is vital: Short periods of unprotected exposure to early morning or late afternoon sun (before 10 AM or after 4 PM) can provide the benefits of vitamin D without significant damage.

Depending on your skin type and location, 15-30 minutes of sun exposure a few times a week is usually enough to maintain healthy vitamin D levels.

Sunscreen Use

Apply sunscreen generously: Use broad-spectrum sunscreen with at least **SPF 30** to protect against UVA (aging) and UVB (burning) rays.

Apply 15 minutes before exposure: Sunscreen takes time to absorb and form a protective barrier.

Reapply every two hours: Sunscreen effectiveness wanes with sweating or swimming. Even if the sunscreen is water-resistant, reapply it after swimming or sweating.

Protective Clothing and Shade

Use **wide-brimmed hats, sunglasses, and long-sleeved clothing** to protect exposed skin. Seek **shade during peak UV hours** (10 AM to 4 PM) to minimize direct sun exposure.

UPF clothing (Ultraviolet Protection Factor) is designed to block UV rays and can provide an additional layer of protection.

Balanced Approach to Vitamin D

You can still get vitamin D while wearing sunscreen. Studies suggest that while sunscreen reduces the amount of UVB reaching the skin, enough is absorbed to maintain vitamin D levels.

Supplements may be helpful, especially in areas with low sunlight or for individuals at risk of deficiency. Always consult with a health-care provider.

Signs of Overexposure

Watch for **redness, tenderness, or peeling** as signs of sun damage.

If you experience sunburn, use **aloe vera** or over-the-counter lotions to soothe the skin and stay out of the sun until healed.

Summary of Balance:

Get **brief sun exposure** (15-30 minutes) during optimal times for vitamin D, but always use sunscreen for extended outdoor activities.

Apply **sunscreen regularly** and combine it with **protective clothing and shade** during peak hours.

Don't rely solely on sunscreen—protection involves a **holistic approach**, including awareness of sun intensity, time of day, and skin care.

This balance allows you to enjoy the health benefits of sunlight while keeping your skin protected and healthy.

Light Therapy Options for Those with Limited Access to Sunlight: Exploring the use of artificial sunlight devices for regions with limited natural light.

For individuals living in regions with limited access to natural sunlight, especially during winter or in high-latitude areas, **light therapy** using artificial sunlight can help compensate for reduced exposure. These devices can improve mood, regulate sleep, and support overall well-being, particularly for conditions like **seasonal affective disorder (SAD)** or **vitamin D deficiency.**

Here's a guide to exploring light therapy options:

Understanding Light Therapy

Light therapy, or phototherapy, involves exposure to **bright, artificial light** that mimics natural sunlight.

It is commonly used to **treat Seasonal Affective Disorder (SAD)**, a type of depression related to seasonal changes. It can also help people with sleep disorders or those who spend little time outdoors.

Types of Light Therapy Devices Light Therapy Lamps (SAD Lamps):

These devices emit **bright light, typically 10,000 lux**, mimicking the intensity of daylight.

Full-spectrum light simulates natural sunlight, often without harmful UV rays.

For practical use, sit near the lamp for about **20-30 minutes daily**, preferably in the morning, to regulate your circadian rhythm and boost your mood.

Light Boxes:

Light boxes offer high-intensity light and are often used to treat mood disorders.

Like light therapy lamps, these should provide around **10,000 lux** and be positioned at eye level or above to replicate the angle of sunlight.

Dawn Simulators:

These devices mimic a natural sunrise by gradually increasing the light in your bedroom as you wake up. This method helps regulate the body's internal clock and improves sleep quality.

Vitamin D Lamps:

Unlike regular light therapy lamps, these emit **UVB rays** that stimulate vitamin D production in the skin, much like natural sunlight. However, these must be used cautiously to avoid skin damage, and it's best to consult a healthcare provider before use.

Benefits of Light Therapy

Mood and Energy Boost: Light therapy effectively combat **Seasonal Affective Disorder (SAD)** and helps boost mood and energy levels during darker months.

Improved Sleep: Regular exposure to bright light can help reset your **circadian rhythm**, making it easier to fall asleep and wake up regularly.

Enhanced Focus and Productivity: Exposure to bright light during the day can improve alertness and focus, particularly in indoor work environments with insufficient natural light.

Choosing the Right Device

Look for devices that offer **10,000 lux** of brightness without UV rays for SAD treatment or other mood disorders

Ensure the light emitted is **full-spectrum white light** (for SAD), or choose UVB light carefully if you are seeking to address vitamin D deficiency.

Devices should have **UV filters** to avoid skin damage, especially for sensitive skin.

How to Use Light Therapy Safely

Timing: Use light therapy in the **morning** to align with your body's natural wake cycle and improve mood throughout the day. Avoid using it too late in the day, as it can interfere with sleep.

Duration: Start with **20-30 minutes** of exposure per day. You can adjust the time based on your response, but avoid excessive exposure as it may cause headaches or eye strain.

Distance from Device: Follow the manufacturer's instructions regarding how far you should sit from the device, usually around **16 to 24 inches**.

Consult a Healthcare Professional: Especially if you have conditions like bipolar disorder, consult your doctor before starting light therapy, as it can sometimes trigger manic episodes.

Additional Benefits for Vitamin D Deficiency

If sunlight is limited in your area, **vitamin D lamps** that emit UVB light can help boost your vitamin D levels. However, these should be used cautiously and according to proper guidelines to avoid skin damage.

Vitamin D supplements may also be an option, as they provide the benefits of sunlight without needing UV exposure

Additional Considerations

Light therapy devices should be **UV-free** unless specified for vitamin D production.

Consider using a **dawn simulator** to help regulate your body's internal clock and improve wakefulness.

Combine light therapy with **short walks** outside, even on cloudy days, for maximum benefit.

Recommended Products:

Verilux HappyLight: A well-known light therapy lamp that provides 10,000 lux for mood improvement.

Circadian Optics Light Therapy Lamp: This compact and portable lamp offers bright, natural light and is UV-free.

NatureBright SunTouch Plus: A popular model that combines light therapy with negative ion therapy for improved mood and energy.

By using artificial sunlight devices, you can effectively combat the effects of limited sunlight, improving mood, regulating sleep, and maintaining overall health.

Mindful Sun Practices: Creating a balanced routine for outdoor activities to maximize sunlight's benefits for both mind and body.

Creating a balanced routine for outdoor activities to maximize sunlight's benefits for both mind and body requires mindful sun practices. These practices help you harness the positive effects of sunlight on mood, energy, and physical health while minimizing risks. Here's how to develop a balanced, sun-conscious approach:

Plan Outdoor Activities Around Optimal Sunlight Times

Morning and Late Afternoon Exposure: Schedule outdoor activities—like walking, gardening, or exercising—during the **early morning (before 10 AM)** or **late afternoon (after 4 PM)**. These times allow you to enjoy the benefits of sunlight without overexposure to harmful UV rays.

Take advantage of natural light to boost **mood** and **energy** levels.

Sunlight helps increase serotonin, which contributes to feelings of happiness and well-being.

Combine Physical Activity with Sunlight

Walking or Hiking: Take short morning walks or hikes in nature to combine exercise with sun exposure. These activities promote cardiovascular health, improve mood, and strengthen the body.

Outdoor Yoga or Meditation: Practice mindfulness exercises like **yoga or meditation** in the early morning sunlight. This routine helps reduce stress, improves focus, and enhances the mind-body connection.

Swimming or Water Activities: If you enjoy water-based activities, plan them in the morning or evening when the sun is less intense. Wear sunscreen and use UV-protective swimwear for added protection.

Incorporate Mindfulness in Sun Practices

Be Present in Nature: Practice mindfulness by fully present and engaging your senses while spending time outside. Focus on the warmth of the sun, the feel of the breeze, or the sounds of nature, which promotes relaxation and reduces stress.

Observe the Light: Pay attention to how sunlight changes throughout the day. Morning light can feel softer and energizing, while evening light offers a calming effect. This awareness helps you connect with the natural rhythm of the day.

Practice Safe Sun Protection

Apply Sunscreen: Use a broad-spectrum sunscreen with **SPF 30 or**

higher, even during morning or evening hours if you're out for extended periods. Apply 15-20 minutes before sun exposure and reapply every two hours.

Wear Protective Clothing: When outdoors, wear **wide-brimmed hats, sunglasses, and long-sleeved clothing** to protect your skin from UV exposure while allowing enough sunlight for health benefits.

Use Shade Strategically: During peak sun hours (10 AM to 4 PM), seek Shade whenever possible or take breaks under trees, umbrellas, or shelters to reduce exposure to direct sunlight.

Incorporate Vitamin D Awareness

While brief, unprotected sun exposure helps your body produce **vitamin D**, limiting this to **15-30 minutes** a few times a week, depending on your skin type and location, is essential.

For those in regions with low sunlight or during winter months, consider **light therapy** devices or **vitamin D supplements** as part of your routine to maintain healthy levels of the vitamin.

Align Sun Exposure with Your Daily Routine

Morning Routine: If possible, **wake up with the sun** and spend 10-20 minutes outside to boost energy and regulate your circadian rhythm. This helps balance hormones like melatonin and cortisol, improving sleep and alertness.

Lunchtime Walk: If your schedule allows, take a quick walk outdoors during midday. Stick to shaded areas or wear proper sun protection to avoid harsh UV rays.

Evening Relaxation: After a busy day, enjoy the calming effect of the late afternoon or evening sun by spending time in a park or on a patio. This is a perfect time for gentle activities like stretching, reading, or socializing with loved ones.

Mind-Body Connection through Nature

Forest Bathing (Shinrin-Yoku): If possible, practice **forest bathing** by walking in wooded areas or green spaces. Exposure to sunlight filtered through trees and the calming natural environment reduces stress, lowers blood pressure, and improves mood.

Gratitude and Reflection: Incorporate moments of **appreciation** during your outdoor activities by reflecting on sunlight and nature's positive effects on your mind and body.

Hydration and Nutrition

Stay Hydrated: Sun exposure can lead to dehydration, especially during physical activities. Carry water and drink regularly to maintain hydration, which is critical to overall wellness and prevents sun-related fatigue.

Consume Antioxidant-Rich Foods: Eat foods high in antioxidants, like berries, leafy greens, and nuts, to help your skin recover from sun exposure and protect against cellular damage caused by UV rays.

Seasonal Adjustments

During winter or cloudy months, maximize time outside whenever there is sunlight. Even overcast days provide some exposure to UV rays, and spending time outdoors can improve mood.

Incorporate **light therapy** if you live in areas with prolonged winter darkness or limited sunlight to maintain healthy circadian rhythms and avoid mood disruptions.

Track Your Time and Exposure

Be mindful of how long you're exposed to the sun. Consider journaling about your outdoor activities and how your mind and body feel afterward. This helps you adjust your routine to suit your health and wellness needs.

Sample Daily Mindful Sun Routine:

1. **Morning (7:00 AM - 8:00 AM):**
15-20 minutes of outdoor yoga or a light walk in the morning sun. Practice deep breathing and mindfulness to start the day with a calm mind.

Midday (12:00 PM – 1:00 PM):

Spend 10-15 minutes in the Shade outdoors, eating lunch or reading.
Protect yourself with sunscreen and a wide-brimmed hat if exposed to direct sunlight.

Evening (5:00 PM – 6:00 PM):

Enjoy a slow-paced walk or relaxation in the late afternoon sun. Reflect on your day while soaking in the calming rays of the evening.

By creating a routine that balances mindful sun exposure with protection, you can harness the benefits of sunlight for both your mental and physical well-being while minimizing potential risks.

Conclusion: Embracing the Healing Power of Sunlight Summary of the Benefits of Sunlight on Holistic Health

Sunlight is a vital force that contributes significantly to our overall health and well-being, influencing us physically, mentally, and emotionally.

Moderate exposure to sunlight offers a wide range of benefits that support holistic health.

Physical Health:

Vitamin D Production: Sunlight stimulates vitamin D production, which is essential for calcium absorption. It promotes strong bones and reduces the risk of osteoporosis and fractures.

Immune System Support: Regular sun exposure enhances the immune system, improving the body's ability to fight infections and reduce inflammation.

Cardiovascular Health: Sunlight has been linked to improved heart health. It can potentially reduce the risk of cardiovascular diseases by lowering blood pressure through the release of nitric oxide.

Mental Well-Being:

Mood Enhancement: Sunlight boosts serotonin levels, which enhances mood, increases energy, and helps prevent depression, including Seasonal Affective Disorder (SAD).

Cognitive Function: Exposure to sunlight, particularly in the morning, regulates circadian rhythms, improving sleep quality and supporting cognitive sharpness, focus, and memory.

Emotional Wellness:

Stress Reduction: Sunlight has a calming effect, reducing stress and promoting relaxation.

Emotional Balance: Sunlight improves sleep, boosts mood, and enhances physical health, helping create emotional stability and balance and contributing to an overall sense of well-being.

In summary, sunlight is a natural and accessible tool that supports the body, mind, and spirit. By incorporating regular, moderate sun exposure into our lives, we can benefit from its holistic contributions to our physical health, mental clarity, and emotional happiness, leading to a healthier and more fulfilling life.

Practical Tips for Daily Sunlight Exposure

Incorporating sunlight into your daily routine is an easy and effective way to improve your overall health and well-being. Here are some practical tips to help you mindfully enjoy the benefits of sunlight while ensuring safety and long-term health gains:

Aim for Morning Sunlight

Morning light is the best time to get your daily dose of sunlight. It's gentle on the skin and helps regulate your **circadian rhythm**, which improves sleep and mental clarity. Try to get outside between **8 a.m. and 10 a.m.** for 15–30 minutes of natural sunlight.

Take Short, Frequent Breaks Outdoors

Instead of spending long periods in the sun, aim for **short, frequent exposure** throughout the day. You can walk during lunch or step outside for a few minutes of fresh air and sunshine during work breaks. This regular exposure helps maintain vitamin D levels and keeps your energy high.

Combine Sunlight with Physical Activity

Engaging in outdoor activities like walking, gardening, cycling, or yoga in the sun provides health benefits from sunlight and physical exercise.

This combination boosts mood, strengthens bones, and supports overall fitness.

Find Sun-Friendly Spots at Home or Work

Create a **sunlight-friendly space** at home or work, such as sitting by a window or in an outdoor area. Even indirect sunlight can have mood-boosting effects. If you have access to a balcony, porch, or garden, make spending time there a regular part of your routine.

Be Mindful of the Time of Day

Avoid prolonged sun exposure between **10 a.m. and 4 p.m.**, when UV rays are the strongest. If you need to be outside during these hours, protect your skin with **sunscreen**, **hats**, or **protective clothing**. This ensures you get the benefits of sunlight without the risk of sunburn or long-term skin damage.

Enjoy Sunlight During Social Activities

Incorporate sunlight into **social events**. Meet friends for outdoor coffee, host picnics, or take family walks in the park. Sharing time outdoors with others improves your physical health and enhances emotional and mental well-being through social connection.

Use Sunlight to Reset Your Sleep Cycle

If you struggle with sleep, expose yourself to **natural light in the morning** to help reset your internal body clock. This simple practice can help regulate your sleep-wake cycle, leading to better sleep quality and increased daytime alertness.

Be Aware of Your Skin Type

Your skin type affects how much sun exposure you need. Those with fair skin may need just **10–15 minutes**, while individuals with darker skin may require **30 minutes or more** to produce adequate vitamin D. Adjust your sun exposure based on your skin's sensitivity.

Consider Seasonal Adjustments

In the winter months or in areas with limited sunlight, you should **increase outdoor time** when possible. If natural sunlight is scarce, consider using **light therapy lamps** to mimic sunlight, especially if you're prone to Seasonal Affective Disorder (SAD).

Balance Sunlight with Sunscreen

Apply **broad-spectrum sunscreen** with an SPF of 30 or higher for more extended periods of sun exposure, especially during peak UV hours. This allows you to balance the benefits of sunlight with the protection needed to keep your skin healthy.

By mindfully incorporating these tips into your routine, you can enjoy the positive effects of sunlight on your health, energy, and mood. Regular, moderate sun exposure can be a simple and powerful tool for long-term physical and emotional well-being.

Final Thoughts on Harnessing Nature's Gift: Recognizing Sunlight as a Natural, Accessible Tool for Boosting Health, Energy, and Happiness

Sunlight is one of nature's most influential and accessible tools for enhancing physical, mental, and emotional well-being. By simply stepping outside and allowing our skin to absorb the sun's rays, we tap into a natural source of health benefits that can improve our daily lives and long-term vitality.

Sunlight plays an essential role in the production of vitamin D, supporting strong bones, a robust immune system, and overall physical resilience. It also helps regulate our circadian rhythms, offering the promise of better sleep and sharper cognitive function. Sunlight also positively influences our mood by stimulating the production of serotonin, which boosts energy levels and helps us feel more connected and happy.

In our modern world, where many of us spend the majority of our time indoors, it's easy to overlook the simple, yet powerful, act of spending time in natural light. However, by making a conscious effort to enjoy regular, moderate sun exposure, we can lead to numerous health improvements and a greater sense of well-being.

By embracing sunlight as part of a balanced lifestyle, we can harness nature's free, readily available gift to enhance our physical health, elevate our mood, and increase our overall quality of life. In moderation, sunlight is a vital component of a healthy, energized, and happy life.

Afterword

As we conclude our exploration of sunlight's impact on health and well-being, it's crucial to reiterate that the balance between sun exposure and skin protection is deeply personal and rooted in science and individual needs. This book has extensively covered the benefits of sunlight—its role in vitamin D production, mood enhancement, and therapeutic relief for skin conditions like psoriasis and eczema. However, we've also stressed the need to be aware of the risks of over-exposure, including sunburn, premature aging, and, most importantly, skin cancer.

What remains clear is that sunlight, while a source of vitality, must be approached with respect. Whether you are someone who enjoys outdoor activities, someone managing a skin condition, or simply looking to improve your overall health, the knowledge shared in this book is designed to empower you to make informed decisions about sun exposure and skin protection.

Throughout these pages, we've highlighted the crucial role of **moderation**—the key to harnessing sunlight's benefits while protecting yourself from harm. Phototherapy, a controlled medical treatment using UV light, has demonstrated how science can safely replicate the sun's healing power. Similarly, practical strategies like wearing sunscreen, using protective clothing, and monitoring the UV index allow us to thoughtfully integrate the sun into our lives.

This journey through the science of sunlight has shown us that embracing the sun's benefits is possible without falling victim to its dangers. Our goal is not to shy away from the sun but to engage with it wisely, fostering a relationship that nurtures our skin and overall well-being.

As you move forward, consider this knowledge a guide—not just for maintaining skin health but for promoting a balanced lifestyle that respects the sun's immense power. Every person's needs are different, and understanding your body and its relationship with sunlight will help you confidently enjoy its warmth and light.

Thank you for joining this journey of discovery. May your path be filled with sunlight and safely enjoyed, and may you continue to explore the wonders of nature with a healthy balance in mind.